T0178018

WHAT'S SO FUNNY?

Humor-Based Activities for Social Skill Development

WHAT'S SO FUNNY?

Humor-Based Activities for Social Skill Development

Rachel Chaiet, MS, OTR/L
Occupational Therapist
Bethel, New York

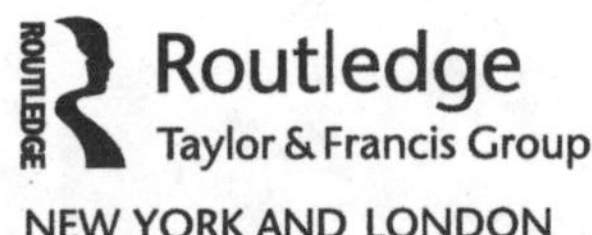

NEW YORK AND LONDON

Rachel Chaiet has no financial or proprietary interest in the materials presented herein.

First published 2022 by SLACK Incorporated

Published 2024 by Routledge
605 Third Avenue, New York, NY 10158

and by Routledge
4 Park Square, Milton Park, Abingdon, Oxon, OX14 4RN

Routledge is an imprint of the Taylor & Francis Group, an informa business

Library of Congress Cataloging-in-Publication Data

Names: Chaiet, Rachel, author.
Title: What's so funny? : humor-based activities for social skill development / Rachel Chaiet.
Description: Thorofare, NJ : SLACK Incorporated, [2022] | Includes bibliographical references and index.
Identifiers: LCCN 2021027389 (print) | ISBN 9781630917203 (paperback)
Subjects: MESH: Autism Spectrum Disorder--therapy | Developmental Disabilities--therapy | Laughter Therapy | Social Skills | BISAC: MEDICAL / Allied Health Services / Occupational Therapy | EDUCATION / Special Education / General
Classification: LCC RC553.A88 (print) | NLM WS 350.8.P4 | DDC 616.85/882--dc23
LC record available at https://lccn.loc.gov/2021027389

Cover Artist: Amarie Mitchell

ISBN: 9781630917203 (pbk)
ISBN: 9781003526933 (ebk)

DOI:10.4324/9781003526933

Dedication

This book is dedicated to Max and Mikaia Rose, for your patience and understanding, and to my mother, Christine, for teaching me how to look at the funny side of everything.

Contents

Dedication . . . . *v*
Acknowledgments . . . . *ix*
About the Author . . . . *xi*
Introduction . . . . *xiii*

Chapter 1 **About This Program** **1**
Intended Audience 1
Intended Participants 1
Benefits of the Program 2
Research-Based Strategies 2

Chapter 2 **Background Information** **5**
Order of Lessons 5
Social-Emotional Development 5
Humor Development 6
Humor Use in Individuals With Developmental Disabilities 7
Teaching Humor 7

Chapter 3 **Physical Comedy: Face and Body** **9**
Lesson 1: Funny Faces 9
Lesson 2: Funny Face Acting 19
Lesson 3: Funny Body 26

Chapter 4 **Physical Comedy: Costumes and Impressions** **35**
Lesson 1: Funny Costumes 35
Lesson 2: Impressions 44

Chapter 5 **Physical Comedy: Slapstick** **53**
Lesson 1: Introduction to Slapstick 53
Lesson 2: Messy Slapstick 65

Chapter 6 **Incongruency** **79**
Lesson 1: Funny Animals 79
Lesson 2: Funny People 87
Lesson 3: Funny Sizes 94

Chapter 7 **Pranks** **101**
Lesson 1: Food Pranks 101
Lesson 2: Water Pranks 106
Lesson 3: Bug Pranks 111
Lesson 4: Gross Pranks 117
Lesson 5: Money Pranks 122

Chapter 8 **Sound and Word Play** **129**
Lesson 1: Sound Effects 129
Lesson 2: Rhyming Words 135

Chapter 9 **Jokes** **143**
Lesson 1: Rhyming Jokes 143
Lesson 2: Homophone Jokes 150
Lesson 3: Silly Sound Jokes 157
Lesson 4: Knock-Knock Jokes 164

Chapter 10 **Three W Questions of Being Funny** **171**
Lesson 1: What Is Funny? 171
Lesson 2: Who Can You Be Funny With? 180
Lesson 3: When Can You Be Funny? 189

Index *197*

Acknowledgments

I would like to thank The Center for Discovery, a wonderful and magical place, for inspiring me to set the bar high for myself and each individual I work with in order to achieve great things.

I also want to acknowledge Jessica Piatak, OTD, OTR/L; Bailee Hymers, MS, OTR/L; Caitlin Bennett, MS Ed, BCBA; and Conio Loretto, MS, LCAT, MT-BC for their assistance and feedback during the development of the various humor-based activities.

Special thanks goes out to all my favorite photograph "models"; my husband, Max Chaiet, for doing all the shooting and editing; and my mother, Christine Thompson, for the illustrations.

About the Author

Rachel Chaiet, MS, OTR/L is an occupational therapist from Bethel, New York who has worked with children and adolescents with developmental disabilities for over 10 years. She obtained her bachelor's and master's degree from Misericordia University in Dallas, Pennsylvania in 2010. She has presented at multiple conferences for the American Occupational Therapy Association, American Speech–Language–Hearing Association, and American Massage Therapy Association alongside her colleagues on humor-based interventions, as well as other interventions to address social participation for individuals with developmental disabilities. She has also published articles in *OT Advance* and *OT Practice* on various interventions related to improving social participation for this population. In her spare time, she can be found "clowning around" with her own young daughter, Mikaia, and husband, Max.

Introduction

I have been a pediatric occupational therapist for 9.5 years, working mostly with individuals ages 13 to 21 years with developmental disabilities. My main objective as an occupational therapist is to help the people on my caseload live enriched and fulfilled lives by maximizing their participation in valued, age-appropriate life activities. For adolescents with developmental disabilities, social participation is one of the key areas I typically address, as making and keeping friends has been shown to be more challenging for this population (Freidman & Rizzolo, 2017). One aspect of social participation that always seemed more challenging for the individuals I was working with was using humor. Over the years, I found that many would attempt to use humor in a variety of ways, but it was typically not used to engage with others and, many times, not the most socially appropriate, such as thinking it was hilarious to push people down or using curse words or talking about private body parts to be funny. Others would find one very specific thing humorous, whether it was a song, a video clip of a show, or a certain toy, and would listen, watch, or talk about that one thing over and over again. These individuals often did not tap into one of the most powerful functions of humor—to make friends. Research has shown that humor is a powerful tool in building relationships, as people naturally want to be around people who make them laugh and feel good (Ziv, 2009). I had an idea—if my students could be taught how to use humor appropriately, it may help them to connect with others and even build friendships.

I started trying out different funny face and slapstick activities during group sessions. I then went to a local dollar store and picked up some inexpensive props: a whoopie cushion, a prank can of nuts with a toy snake that pops out, some silly glasses and teeth, and others, and brought them in. It was very exciting to see that, sure enough, many students found these "humor-based activities" enjoyable and motivating. It also created a fun way to discuss and practice appropriate facial expressions and body language. I noticed that by structuring the activities and using physical props, many of my students were finding it easier to engage with their classmates and even smiling and/or laughing with them. From there, I began to look into ways to continue to expand their humor skills and to help them understand what is funny versus what is considered inappropriate. Before I knew it, I had built up my own repertoire of activities and strategies that I am now able to share with you in this book.

I hope that you are able to find some of the same success with the students, clients, or loved ones that you try these activities with. My wish is for humor to be used as both a means and an end to improve their social interaction skills and, ultimately, strengthen their connection with the people around them.

—Rachel Chaiet, MS, OTR/L

CHAPTER 1

About This Program

Intended Audience

This program can be used by professionals who work with individuals with developmental disabilities and address social participation within their intervention or educational sessions, including but not limited to occupational therapists, speech-language pathologists, special education teachers, and psychologists. In addition, caregivers and other paraprofessionals may also benefit from using these strategies to improve the social skills of those who have challenges in this area. Lessons can be used in both a group or individual format with either their peers or family members.

Intended Participants

This program was designed for individuals ages 7 years to adult with developmental disabilities, such as autism, Down syndrome, attention deficit hyperactivity disorder, or others that affect their social participation skills. Participants may have a wide functional range of abilities, including but not limited to:

- Individuals who appear to have a very limited concept of humor or basic developmental level of humor
- Individuals who need to improve their understanding of socially appropriate humor (e.g., what is funny vs. what is cruel)
- Individuals who need to work on appropriate use of humor (i.e., when and when not to use humor)
- Individuals who are nonverbal with very limited expressive communication skills or use augmentative communication devices
- Individuals who have a difficult time initiating social interactions with their peers

Chaiet, R. *What's So Funny?: Humor-Based Activities for Social Skill Development* (pp. 1-4).

Although this program has been created for individuals with limitations of social, communicative, and emotional expression skills, participants do need to have some prerequisite skills in order to optimally benefit from all of the activities, including:

- Ability to visually attend to the instructor, other participants, and him- or herself in a mirror
- Ability to visually attend to materials used
- Ability to sustain attention to the task for at least 5 to 10 minutes at a time (breaks can be provided, if needed)
- Ability to imitate basic movements of the face
- Ability to follow basic directions
- Ability to imitate various gross motor movements
- Demonstrates basic fine motor skills to activate some of the pranks
- Ability to use a form of expressive communication (verbal, communication device, communication board, activate switches, etc.)

Benefits of the Program

The main objective of this program is to use the universal tool of humor to help participating individuals with developmental disabilities increase their social interaction and engagement with others. Since it is key to be aware of a person's emotions and to react accordingly with one's own emotions in order to successfully interact with others, emphasis is also placed on improving one's ability to identify and use facial expressions and body language. An added benefit may be to help participants begin to develop or expand their repertoire of humor skills. Each humor-based lesson is easy to facilitate and consists of fun and motivating hands-on activities that have been adapted to make them accessible to individuals with varying levels of function. The supplies required are affordable and can be easily purchased at a local store or through the internet.

Research-Based Strategies

Explicit Instruction

Each lesson in this program is accompanied by a social narrative that uses the technique of explicit instruction, a strategy that has proven effective for teaching various academic and social skills to people with autism spectrum disorders and other developmental disabilities (Braun et al., 2017). Each humor-based activity is introduced and an explanation is given as to what makes it funny. Then, the activity is broken down step-by-step and includes an opportunity to use it to engage with others. The entire narrative uses simple, clear language with pictures in order to improve comprehension for nonreaders and those with cognitive limitations. Instructors are then encouraged to model each activity and provide feedback on each individual's participation.

Seven Humor Habits Program

Another research-based strategy that is integrated into these humor-based lessons are Paul McGhee's Seven Humor Habits Program, which include "surround yourself with humor, cultivate a playful attitude, laugh more often, create your own verbal humor, look for humor in daily life, laugh at yourself, and find humor in the midst of stress" (Ruch et al., 2018, p. 3). Practicing these habits has been found to help increase a person's ability to use humor with others, as well as increase overall positive emotions and life satisfaction. By exposing the participants to a variety of different types of humor regularly, they are being surrounded by humor and encouraged to laugh more often. Facilitators have an important role in ensuring they demonstrate each of the activities with high energy and enthusiasm in order to create an environment of playfulness. The physical humor sections require participants to make funny faces and body movements, wear silly costumes, and participate in crazy scenarios, which gives them the opportunity to laugh at themselves. The Sound Effects and Rhyming Words lessons encourage participants to make their own verbal humor by having them come up with their own humorous sounds and rhyming phrases.

Social Interaction Motor Planning Exercises Intervention

Emotional reciprocity, or the ability to attend to the emotional cues of others and respond appropriately with your own emotional expressions, is key to developing appropriate social interaction skills (Molnar-Szakacs et al., 2009). Research has shown that individuals with autism, Down syndrome, and other developmental disabilities often have difficulty with emotional reciprocity as they may find it challenging to interpret and/or use facial expressions, which affects their ability to interact and build friendships with others (Wishart et al., 2007). In addition to difficulty with reading and using appropriate facial expressions, individuals with certain developmental disabilities, such as autism, may have difficulty with understanding and using appropriate body language (U.S. Department of Health and Human Services et al., 2016).

The Social Interaction Motor Planning Exercises (SIMPLE) intervention strategies consist of using sensory-motor and role-playing activities to increase awareness of the emotions connected to universal facial expressions and body language (Gutman et al., 2015). Facilitators are encouraged to provide verbal, gestural, and touch prompts, as needed, to increase an individual's awareness of his or her own facial expressions. In many of the physical comedy lessons of this program, participants are encouraged to try various facial expressions and body movements and identify expressions and movements of others to improve their ability to label what emotions are being conveyed. In addition, verbal, gestural, and touch feedback is encouraged to be given to the participants in order to improve their emotional reciprocity skills.

References

Braun, G., Austin, C., & Ledbetter-Cho, K. (2017). *Practice guide: Explicit instruction in reading comprehension for students with autism spectrum disorder.* U.S. Department of Education, Office of Special Education Program.

Gutman, S., Raphael-Greenfield, R., & Rao, A. (2012). Effect of a motor-based role-play intervention on the social behaviors of adolescents with high-functioning autism: Multiple-baseline single-subject design. *American Journal of Occupational Therapy, 66*(5), 529-537.

Molnar-Szakacs, I., Wang, M., Laugeson, E., Overy, K., Wu, W., & Piggot, J. (2009). Autism, emotion recognition and the mirror neuron system: The case of music. *McGill Journal of Medicine, 12*(2), 87.

Ruch, W., Hofmann, J., Rusch, S., & Stolz, H. (2018). Training the sense of humor with the 7 Humor Habits Program and satisfaction with life. *HUMOR: International Journal of Humor Research, 31*(2), 287-309.

U.S. Department of Health and Human Services, National Institutes of Health, National Institute of Deafness and Other Communication Disorders. (2016). *Autism spectrum disorder: Communication problems in children.* (NIH Publication No. 97-4315). https://www.nidcd.nih.gov/health/autism-spectrum-disorder-communication-problems-children

Wishart, J., Cebula, K., Willis, D., & Pitcairn, T. (2007). Understanding of facial expressions of emotion by children with intellectual disabilities of differing aetiology. *Journal of Intellectual Disability Research, 51*(7), 551-563.

CHAPTER 2

Background Information

Order of Lessons

Since social-emotional skills are essential in order to appropriately use humor to interact with others, the order of the lessons in this book are based on a developmental progression of both humor and social-emotional development. Each subsequent lesson builds off the skills learned in the one before it, so it is ideal to use them in the order in which they are presented. Because this program has been created with individuals of varying abilities in mind, the first lessons are based on a young social-emotional and humor developmental age level of 6 to 12 months. The final lessons are based on a social-emotional and humor developmental level of 7 to 11 years of age. Despite this, a determined effort has been made to make each lesson appropriate for any chronological age.

Social-Emotional Development

At the time a typical-developing child is born, he or she is able to use facial expressions to show anger, fear, and joy. Newborns rely on their caregiver to help them regulate their emotions by providing them with what they need, as they are physically unable to meet their needs themselves (Malik & Marwaha, 2019). The first social exchange is gazing back at the caregiver, soon followed by a smile at 1 to 2 months of age when the caregiver is looking him or her in the eyes and speaking softly. The child begins to vocalize around 4 months, which allows the first dialogue to take place between the child and the caregiver (Malik & Marwaha, 2019). By 8 months, a child will begin to attend to the same things as his or her caregiver by looking at what the caregiver is looking at. At 12 months, a child will begin to point to items he or she wants, and by 18 months, a child will begin to be able to go and get the items he or she wants to share it with

REVIEW QUESTIONS: FUNNY FACE ACTING

Name:______________________________

1. When you sneeze, you say __________.
   A. "WOOHOO!"
   B. "AAAA-CHOO!"
   C. "PEE-YOU!"

2. Look at this person's face. What is she doing?
   A. Smelling something stinky
   B. Sneezing
   C. Sleeping

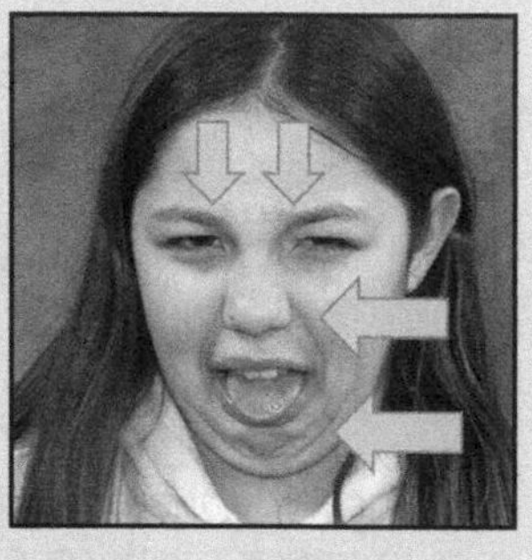

3. When you wake a person up from sleeping and he or she is surprised, the eyebrows will go _______ and the mouth will __________.
   A. Up, close shut
   B. Down, open wide
   C. Up, open wide

4. Look at this person's face. What is she doing?
   A. Smelling something stinky
   B. Sneezing
   C. Sleeping

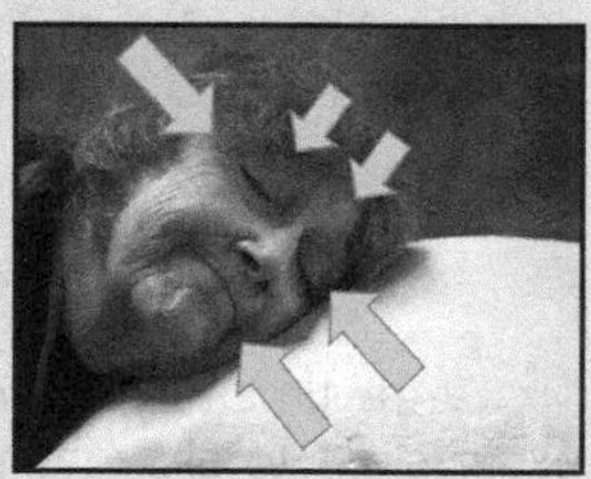

5. What was your favorite thing to act out today? Act it out in the mirror.

Funny Face Acting Review Questions Answer Key

1. B
2. A
3. C
4. C
5. No wrong answer

including teasing and pranks (Buijzen & Valkenburg, 2004). Lastly, in Stage 5, children begin to have a better understanding of how words can have multiple meanings and begin to effectively use riddles and jokes.

Humor Use in Individuals With Developmental Disabilities

Appropriate development of humor does not always come so easy for individuals with a disability compared to their typical-developing peers (Chadwick & Platt, 2018). Someone with an autism spectrum disorder, Down syndrome, or another disorder affecting cognition and/or social intelligence may have a difficult time developing a sense of humor along the same timeline. Difficulty with recognizing and using appropriate facial expressions and body language would affect a child's ability to find incongruity in the silly faces of his or her mom or dad at a young age. Cognitive limitations make it more challenging to understand why slapstick is funny vs. injurious. Expressive and receptive communication challenges may prevent a person from telling or understanding jokes.

Despite these hurdles, a systematic review of the research published in 2018 has concluded that many people with intellectual disabilities do appreciate and utilize humor and proved that it was key in their social interactions (Chadwick & Platt, 2018). Even individuals with an autism spectrum disorder, who often have a specifically challenging time with social interactions, have been shown to have "great enjoyment in socially shared affective experiences of humor" (Southam, 2005, p. 112).

Teaching Humor

For those individuals who do not currently utilize humor, studies have shown that humor is in fact "trainable and training humor leads to desirable outcomes" (Ruch & McGhee, 2014, p. 190). It has been suggested that with the appropriate selection and adaptation of humor-based activities, even those with social skill limitations, such as individuals with developmental disabilities, may be able to "progress through the humor stages" (Southam, 2005, p. 116). Another article concluded that when a person is given positive reinforcement while being humorous, he or she will be encouraged to be humorous again (Lyon, 2006). McGhee concluded from his research that humor can be developed specifically by practicing his Seven Humor Habits Program (Goldstein & Ruch, 2018). In conclusion, there is literature to support teaching humor to individuals with developmental disabilities in order to improve their social participation skills and overall quality of life.

References

Buijzen, M., & Valkenburg, P. (2004). Developing a typology of humor in audiovisual media. *Media Psychology, 6*, 147-167.

Cunningham, J. (2004). Children's humor. In W. G. Scarlett (Ed.), *Children's play* (pp. 93-109). Sage Publications, Inc.

Chadwick, D., & Platt, T. (2018). Investigating humor in social interaction in people with intellectual disabilities: A systematic review of the literature. *Frontiers in Psychology, 9*, 1745.

Goldstein, J., & Ruch, W. (2018). Paul McGhee and humor research. *Humor, 31*(2), 169-181.

Lyon, C. (2006). Humour and the young child: A review of the research literature. *Televizion, 19*, 4-6.

Malik, F., & Marwaha, R. (2019). *Developmental stages of social emotional development in children*. StatPearls Publishing.

Ruch, W., & McGhee, P. (2014). Humor intervention programs. In A. C. Parks & S. Schueller (Eds.), *Wiley-Blackwell handbook of positive psychological interventions* (pp. 179-194). Wiley-Blackwell.

Semrud-Clikeman, M., & Glass, K. (2010). The relation of humor and child development: Social, adaptive and emotional aspects. *Journal of Child Neurology, 25*(10), 1248-1260.

Southam, M. (2005). Humor development: An important cognitive and social skill in the growing child. *Pediatrics, 25*(1), 105-117.

CHAPTER 3

Physical Comedy

Face and Body

Lesson 1: Funny Faces

Objectives

The participant may:

- Improve ability to read someone's emotions by looking at his or her facial expressions
- Improve ability to use facial expressions to express his or her own emotions
- Understand how a person can use his or her facial expressions to be funny and interact with others

Background

In the first stage of social-emotional development, a baby learns to connect with his or her caregivers through looking at their faces and will begin to observe their emotions, as well as display his or her own emotions using universal facial expressions (Malik & Marwaha, 2019). As the child's sense of humor is first developing, he or she often has a "strong preference for visual and physical humor," starting with the funny faces of his or her caregivers (Buijzen & Valkenburg, 2004). Whether they are conscious of this fact, this is why parents will often make funny faces at their babies and toddlers; it often makes them smile, coo, and giggle. Based on social learning theory, which says that humans develop social skills through repeatedly observing and imitating others, this lesson allows for practice of facial expressions to improve the participants' emotional interpretation and expression skills, as well as introduce participants to the concept of using silly faces to be funny and interact with others (Gutman et al., 2012).

Materials

- Funny Faces Visual Story
- Review Questions and Answer Key
- Name That Emotion Cards and Guessing Card
- Handheld mirror

Preparation

- Use the book or photocopy and staple together the visual story entitled Funny Faces
- Photocopy Review Questions, one for each participant
- Photocopy and cut out Name That Emotion cards (can be laminated to increase durability)

Procedure

- Read the visual story to the participants or have them take turns reading each page. When there are questions, be sure to engage the participants and allow them to answer using their specific mode of communication (speech, communication device, sign language, gestures, etc.).
- When introducing each facial expression, first show them by modeling it. Be sure to exaggerate the expressions.
- Encourage participants to look in the mirror each time they are asked to make a facial expression to provide them with visual feedback of the face they are making. If they appear to have difficulty with awareness of the different parts of their face, the instructor can provide a touch prompt to that area of the face or use hand-over-hand assistance to use the participant's hand to touch that part of his or her face. If doing this activity with a group, encourage participants to look at the faces their peers are making.
- After the story is read, play Name That Emotion by having participants take turns picking a card and moving their eyebrows/mouth to act out the emotion or silly face that is on the card. The rest of the participants/instructor guess which emotion or if it is a silly face. The Guessing Card can be used to help participants guess, if they benefit from having choices to answer questions.
- Follow up the activity by having each participant answer the Review Questions, providing assistance as needed. After the participant(s) has completed the questions, the answers given can be compared with the Answer Key.

- Extension activities for this lesson could be:
    - Showing the participants video clips of people expressing different emotions, asking them to identify those emotions and then asking how they can tell
    - Showing the participants video clips of comedians or actors who use exaggerated facial expressions to be funny (e.g., Jim Carrey, Will Ferrell, Mr. Bean)

References

Buijzen, M., & Valkenburg, P. (2004). Developing a typology of humor in audiovisual media. *Media Psychology, 6*, 147-167.

Gutman, S., Raphael-Greenfield, R., & Rao, A. (2012). Effect of a motor-based role-play intervention on the social behaviors of adolescents with high-functioning autism: Multiple-baseline single-subject design. *American Journal of Occupational Therapy, 66*(5), 529-537.

Malik, F., & Marwaha, R. (2019). *Developmental stages of social emotional development in children.* StatPearls Publishing.

EXERCISE: FUNNY FACES

Today, we are going to talk about using your face to show how you feel and to be funny.

You can tell how someone is feeling by looking at his or her eyebrows and mouth. A person's eyebrows show how he or she feels by moving in different directions.

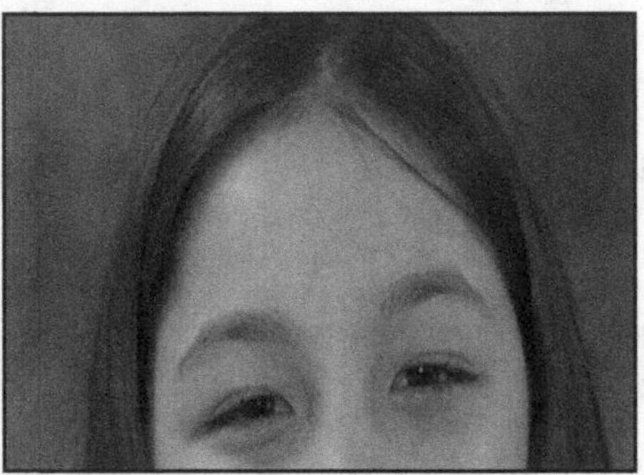

Happy Eyebrows Are Relaxed

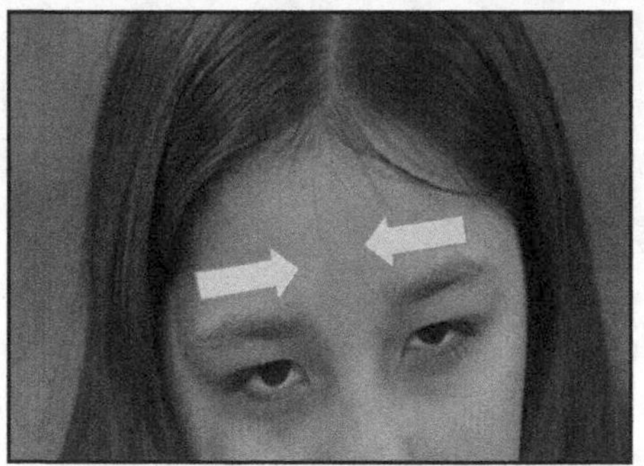

Sad Eyebrows Move in Toward Each Other

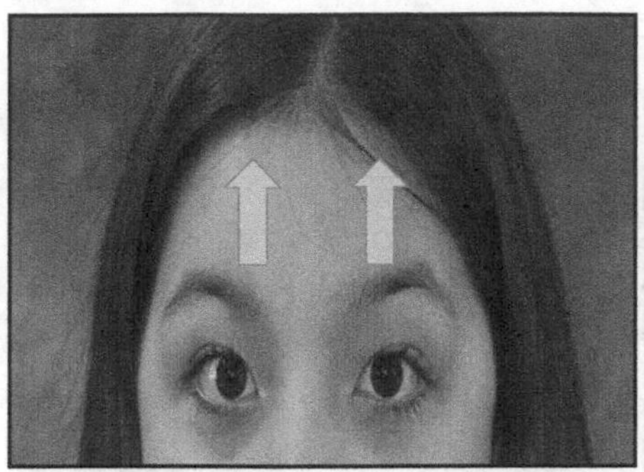

Surprised Eyebrows Move Up

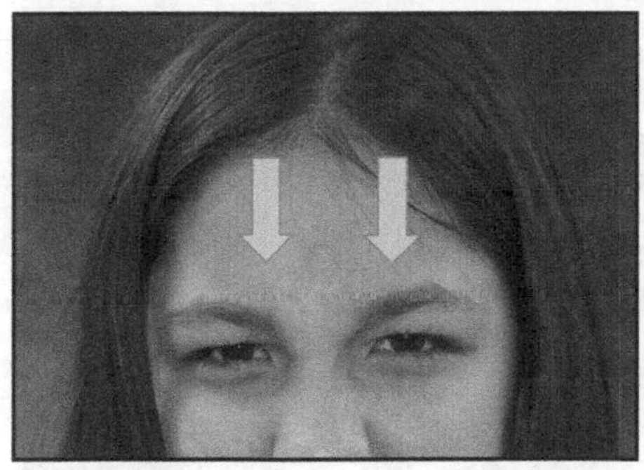

Angry Eyebrows Move Down

Try to show all the different emotions with your eyebrows while looking into the mirror!

A person's mouth can show how he or she feels by making different shapes.

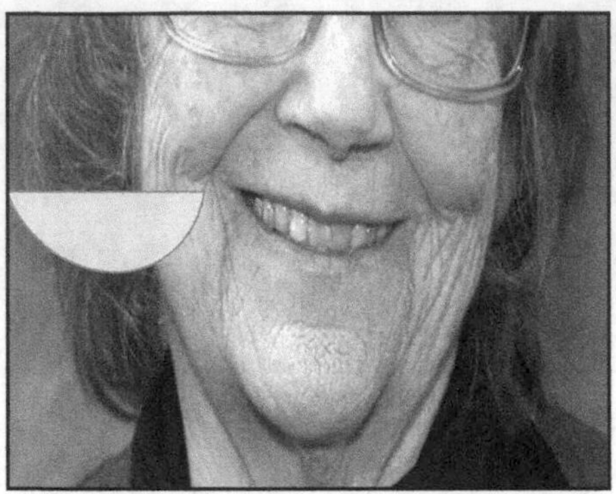

A Happy Mouth Makes a Half Circle

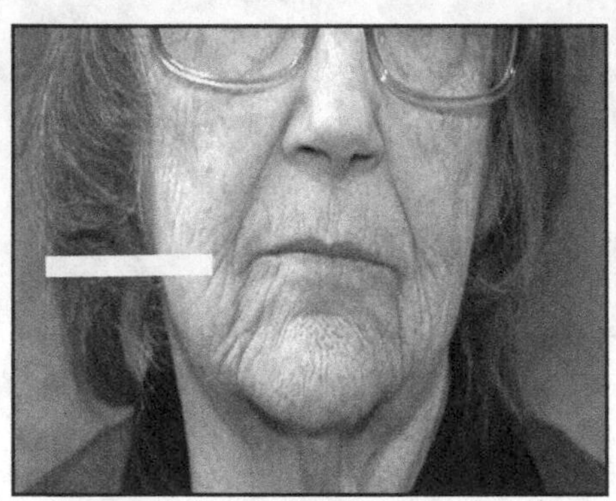

A Sad Mouth Makes a Straight Line

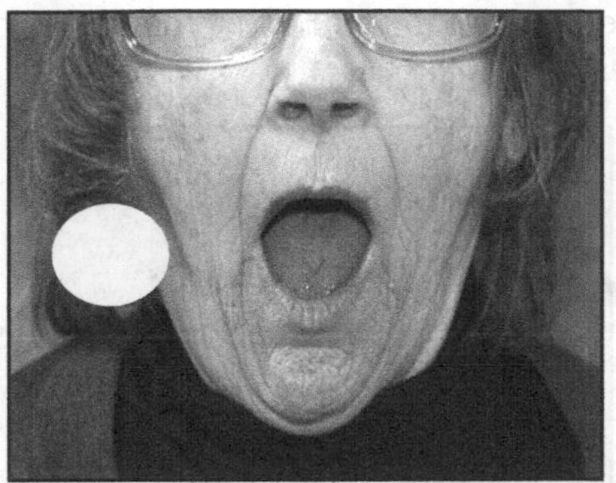

A Surprised Mouth Makes a Circle

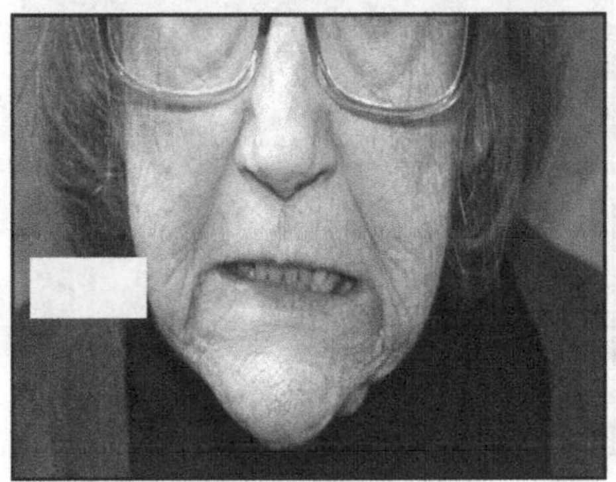

An Angry Mouth Makes a Rectangle

Try to show all different emotions with your mouth while looking into the mirror!

You can also use your face to be funny by moving your eyebrows, mouth, tongue, and nose to make faces.

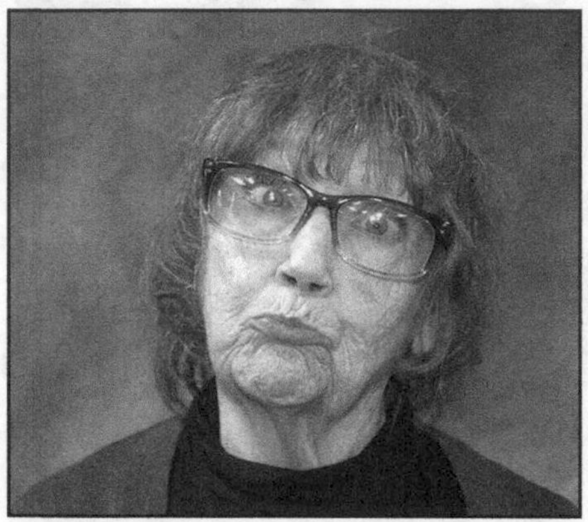

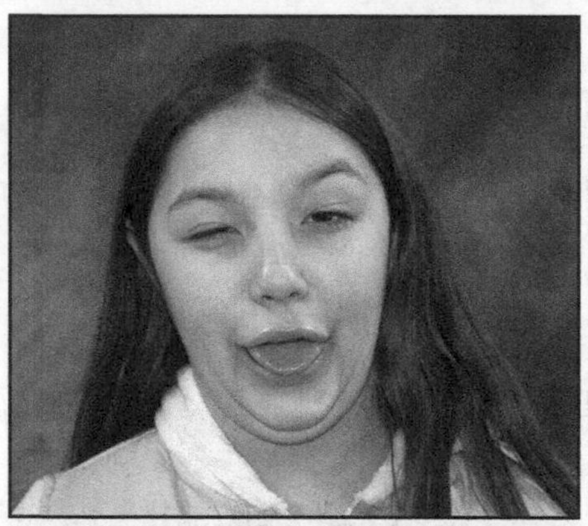

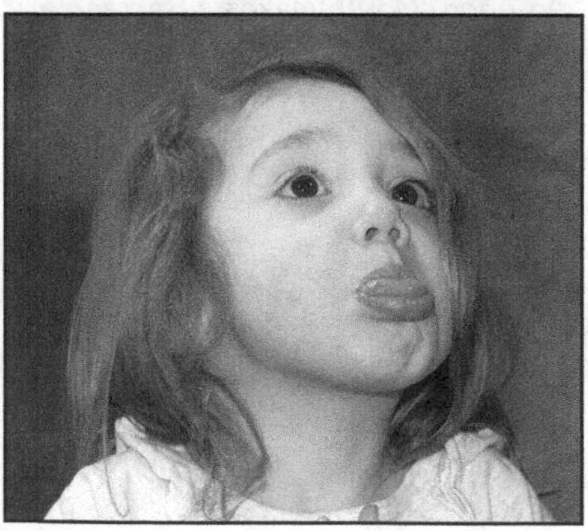

Try to make funny faces with all parts of your face while looking into the mirror!

ACTIVITY: FUNNY FACES

- Take turns picking a card.
- Act out the emotion or silly face that is on the card.
- Have the person(s) guess which emotion you are acting out or if it is a silly face.

Name That Emotion Cards

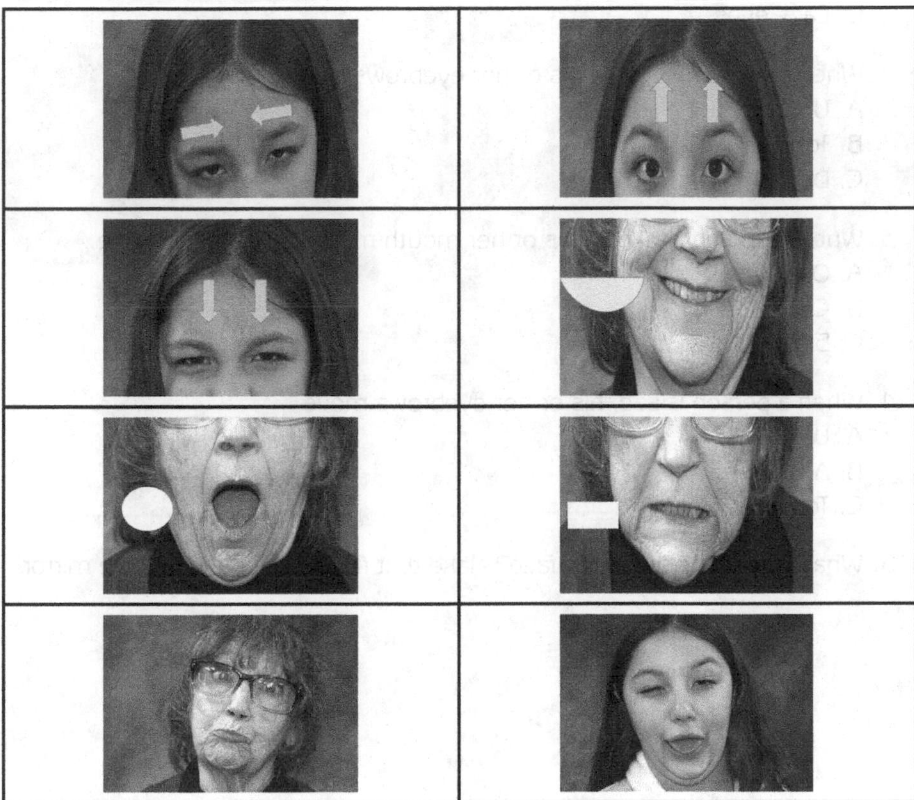

Guessing Card

Happy	**Surprised**
Sad	**Funny Face**
Angry	**I Don't Know**

REVIEW QUESTIONS: FUNNY FACES

Name: ______________________________

1. You can tell how a person is feeling by looking at his or her ______ and ______.
   A. Nose, mouth
   B. Eyebrows, mouth
   C. Ears, eyes

2. When a person is angry, his or her eyebrows go _______.
   A. Up
   B. Together
   C. Down

3. When a person is happy, his or her mouth makes a(n) _____ shape.
   A. Oval
   B. Crescent
   C. Square

4. When a person is sad, his or her eyebrows move ___________.
   A. Up
   B. Apart
   C. Together

5. What is your favorite funny face? Make that face while looking in the mirror.

Funny Faces Review Questions Answer Key

1. B
2. C
3. B
4. C
5. No wrong answer

Lesson 2: Funny Face Acting

Objectives

The participant may:

- Improve ability to read someone's emotions by looking at his or her facial expressions in a specific contextual situation
- Improve ability to use facial expressions to express his or her own emotions in a specific contextual situation
- Use an object to engage in a basic interaction with the instructor or peer
- Understand additional and more complex ways a person can use facial expressions and objects to be funny and interact with others

Background

This lesson builds off of the same skills used in the first, but adds simple, motor-based role-playing activities to draw awareness to the facial expressions used in common scenarios and to practice using those expressions (Gutman et al., 2012). The familiar scenarios used, such as sneezing, smelling a stinky sock, and sleeping/being woken up, are activities that are physical and visual in nature and can be viewed as humorous when exaggerated movements and sounds are used to act them out. The next stage of social-emotional development after reading and using facial expressions is using an object or gestures to interact with another (Malik & Marwaha, 2019). The scenarios in this lesson require these basic interactions, as the instructor or a peer has to pass the participant a sock, tickle his or her nose with a feather, and tap him or her on the shoulder.

Materials

- Funny Face Acting Visual Story
- Review Questions and Answer Key
- Handheld mirror
- Feather
- Small Pillow
- Sock

Preparation

- Use the book or photocopy and staple together the visual story entitled Funny Face Acting
- Photocopy Review Questions, one for each participant

Procedure

- Read the visual story to the participants or have them take turns reading each page. When there are questions, be sure to engage the participants and allow them to answer using their specific mode of communication (speech, communication device, sign language, gestures, etc.).
- When introducing each scenario, first show them by modeling it. Be sure to use exaggerated movements and sounds.
- Encourage participants to look in the mirror each time they are asked to act out a scenario to provide them with visual feedback of the faces they are making. If they appear to have difficulty with awareness of the different parts of their face, the instructor can provide a touch prompt to that area of the face or use hand-over-hand assistance to use the participant's hand to touch that part of his or her face.
- When acting out the scenario, if a participant is nonverbal and does not have a communication device or switch to say the funny phrases, the speaking portion can just be omitted.
- If doing this activity with a group, encourage participants to look at the faces their peers are making and reflect on which emotion they are expressing and/or if they think the face is funny.
- Follow up the activity by having each participant answer the Review Questions, providing assistance as needed. After the participant(s) has completed the questions, the answers given can be compared with the Answer Key.
- Extension activities for this lesson could be:
    - Showing the participants funny video clips or GIFs found on the internet of "silly sneezes," "stinky sock," or "surprise wake-up," asking them to identify what the people are doing in those videos/GIFs and then asking how they can tell

References

Gutman, S., Raphael-Greenfield, R., & Rao, A. (2012). Effect of a motor-based role-play intervention on the social behaviors of adolescents with high-functioning autism: Multiple-baseline single-subject design. *American Journal of Occupational Therapy, 66*(5), 529-537.

Malik, F., & Marwaha, R. (2019). *Developmental stages of social emotional development in children.* StatPearls Publishing.

EXERCISE: FUNNY FACE ACTING

Today, we are going to talk about using your face to act out funny situations! You can move your eyebrows, mouth, and other parts of your face to show how a person would act in a funny situation.

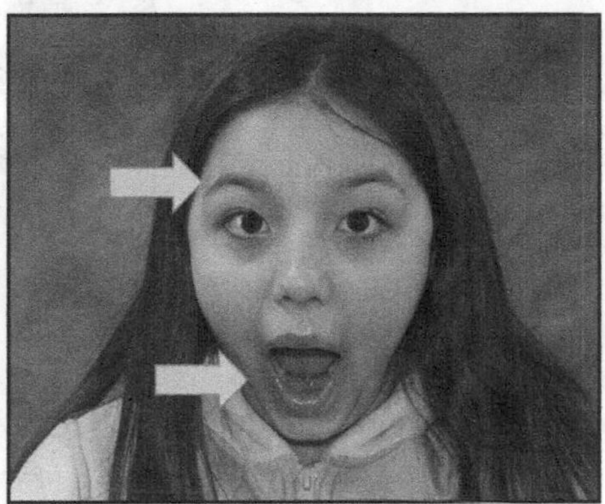

First, we are going to try "Stinky Sock"

When someone hands you a sock, you are going to smell it; use big, silly faces; and say "PEE-YOU!" to pretend it is very stinky!

What Does Your Face Do When You Smell Something Stinky?

- Eyebrows down
- Wrinkle nose
- Stick tongue out
- Say: "PEE-YOU!"

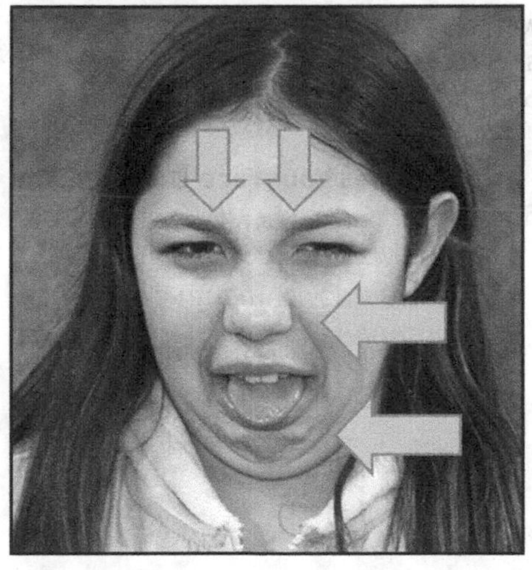

Let's Act Out "Stinky Sock"

- Instructor/peer hands you a sock
- Smell the sock
- Your eyebrows go down, you wrinkle your nose, you stick out your tongue, and say "PEE-YOU!"

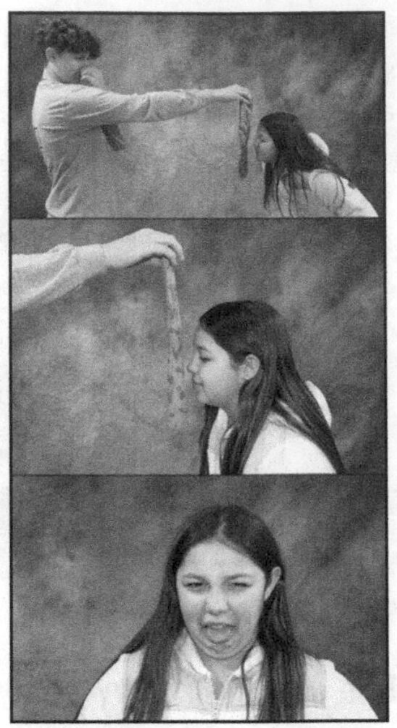

Was It Funny?

- Try smelling the stinky sock in front of a mirror. Is it funny to watch your face make big, silly movements as you say "PEE-YOU!"?
- Watch someone else pretend to smell a stinky sock. Is it funny to watch his or her face make big, silly movements?

Next, we are going to try "Big Sneeze"

When someone tickles your nose with a feather, you are going to use big, silly faces and a loud "AAAA-CHOO!" to pretend you are sneezing!

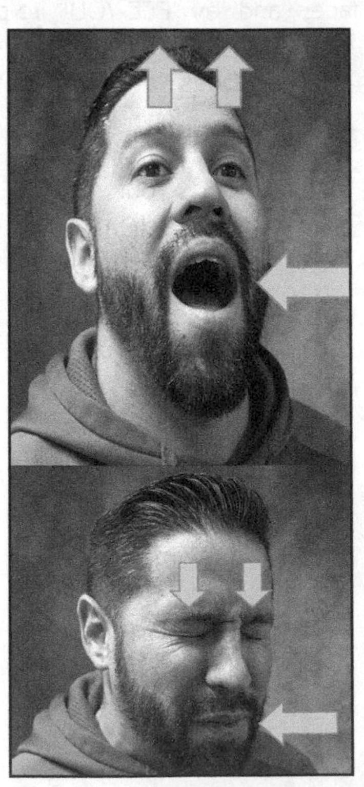

What Does Your Face Do When You Sneeze?

- Eyebrows up, mouth open
- Eyebrows down, mouth closes
- Say: "AAAA-CHOO!"

Let's Act Out "Big Sneeze"

- Instructor/peer tickles your nose with a feather
- Your eyebrows go up and your mouth opens as you say "AAAA-!"
- Your eyebrows go down and your mouth closes as you say "CHOO!"

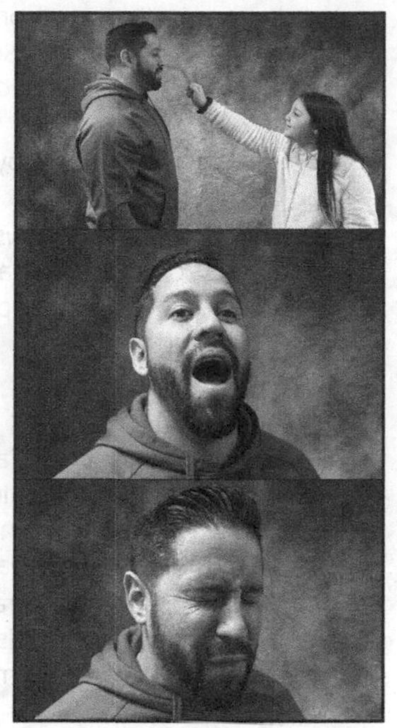

Was It Funny?

- Try your big sneeze in front of a mirror. Is it funny to watch your face make big, silly movements as you say "AAAA-CHOO!"?
- Watch someone else do a pretend big sneeze. Is it funny to watch his or her face make big, silly movements?

Last, we are going to try "Wake Up"

First, you are going to pretend to sleep and snore. Then, someone is going to wake you up and you are going to make big, silly faces as you wake up.

What Does Your Face Look Like When You Sleep?

- Eyebrows rested
- Eyes closed
- Closed mouth
- Say: "ZZZZZZZ!"

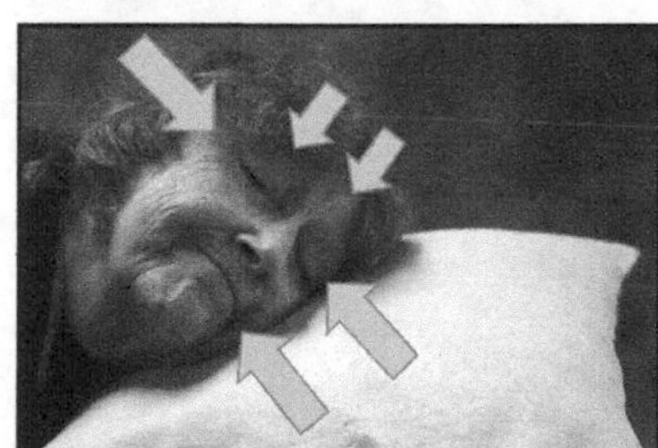

What Does Your Face Look Like if Someone Wakes You Up by Surprise?

- Eyebrows up
- Eyes wide open
- Mouth wide open
- Say: "AHHHHHH!"

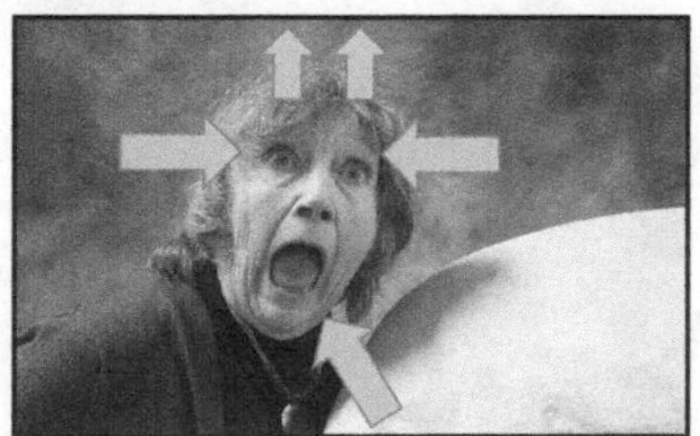

Let's Act Out "Wake Up"

- You lay on a pillow and pretend to sleep with eyebrows relaxed, eyes closed, and mouth closed as you say "ZZZZZZZ!"
- Someone wakes you up by tapping you on the shoulder
- You sit up, your eyebrows go up, your eyes open wide, and your mouth is wide open in surprise. You say "AHHHHHH!"

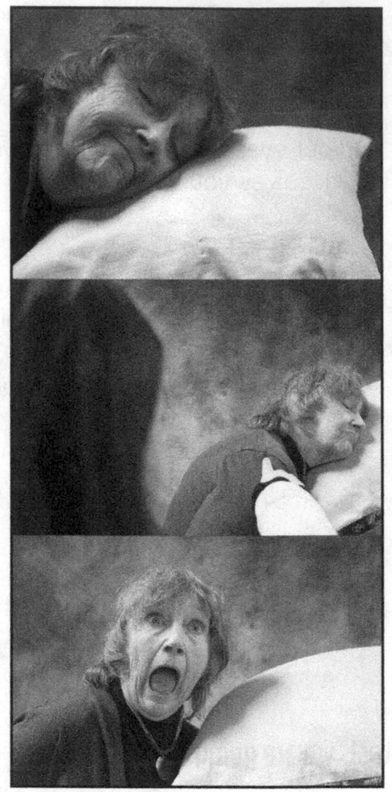

Was It Funny?

- Try pretending to sleep and then wake up in front of a mirror. Is it funny to watch your face make big, silly movements as you wake up?
- Watch someone else pretend to sleep and then wake up. Is it funny to watch his or her face make big, silly movements?

REVIEW QUESTIONS: FUNNY FACE ACTING

Name: ______________________________

1. When you sneeze, you say __________.
   A. "WOOHOO!"
   B. "AAAA-CHOO!"
   C. "PEE-YOU!"

2. Look at this person's face. What is she doing?
   A. Smelling something stinky
   B. Sneezing
   C. Sleeping

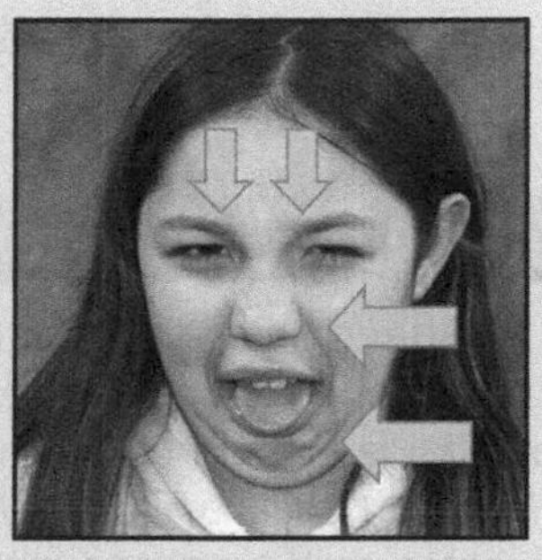

3. When you wake a person up from sleeping and he or she is surprised, the eyebrows will go _______ and the mouth will ___________.
   A. Up, close shut
   B. Down, open wide
   C. Up, open wide

4. Look at this person's face. What is she doing?
   A. Smelling something stinky
   B. Sneezing
   C. Sleeping

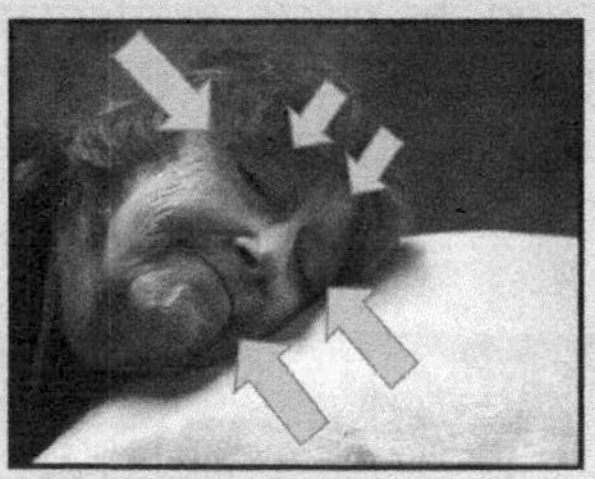

5. What was your favorite thing to act out today? Act it out in the mirror.

Funny Face Acting Review Questions Answer Key

1. B
2. A
3. C
4. C
5. No wrong answer

Lesson 3: Funny Body

Objectives

The participant may:

- Improve ability to read someone's emotions by looking at his or her body language
- Improve ability to use body language to express his or her own emotions
- Understand how a person can use his or her body to be funny and interact with others

Background

After children become more proficient with facial expressions and gain more control of their gross motor movements, gestures are used more effectively alongside eye contact with the caregiver in order to express wants and needs (Malik & Marwaha, 2019). In this lesson, we first take a look at how people can express their emotions with certain postures, arm movements, and leg movements in order to gain practice at using and reading body language. Then, big, funny movements are practiced, as "vigorous arm and leg movements" are perceived as humorous by someone with a developing sense of humor (Buijzen & Valkenburg, 2004). The reason for this is because this behavior is incongruent with a person's typical movement (Semrud-Clikeman & Glass, 2010). Developmentally, this is when games like Peek-a-boo and Pat-a-cake are enjoyed, as quick, exaggerated, and unexpected body gestures are used to engage with the child (Malik & Marwaha, 2019). This lesson affords participants the opportunity to understand and practice using body movements to be funny and interact with others.

Materials

- Funny Body Visual Story
- Review Questions and Answer Key
- Full-length mirror

Preparation

- Use the book or photocopy and staple together the visual story entitled Funny Body
- Photocopy Review Questions, one for each participant

Procedure

- Read the visual story to the participants or have them take turns reading each page. When there are questions, be sure to engage the participants and allow them to answer using their specific mode of communication (speech, communication device, sign language, gestures, etc.).
- When introducing each body movement, first show them by modeling it. Be sure to use exaggerated movements.
- Encourage participants to look in the mirror each time they are asked to make a body movement to provide them with visual feedback of the body language they are using.
- If doing this activity with a group, encourage participants to look at the body movements of their peers.
- Follow up the activity by having each participant answer the Review Questions, providing assistance as needed. After the participant(s) has completed the questions, the answers given can be compared with the Answer Key.
- Extension activities for this lesson could be:
    - Showing the participants video clips of funny mimes who use their body to be funny without speaking, asking them to identify what parts of the body they are using to be funny

References

Buijzen, M., & Valkenburg, P. (2004). Developing a typology of humor in audiovisual media. *Media Psychology, 6*, 147-167.

Malik, F., & Marwaha, R. (2019). *Developmental stages of social emotional development in children*. StatPearls Publishing.

Semrud-Clikeman, M., & Glass, K. (2010). The relation of humor and child development: Social, adaptive and emotional aspects. *Journal of Child Neurology, 25*(10), 1248-1260.

EXERCISE: FUNNY BODY

Besides the face, people use other parts of their body to show emotion and to be funny!

People use their hands/arms to show their emotions.

- Raise your arms and spread out your fingers to show you are excited.
- Clench your fists and hold them in front of you to show you are angry.
- Cover your face with your hands like you are crying to show you are sad.

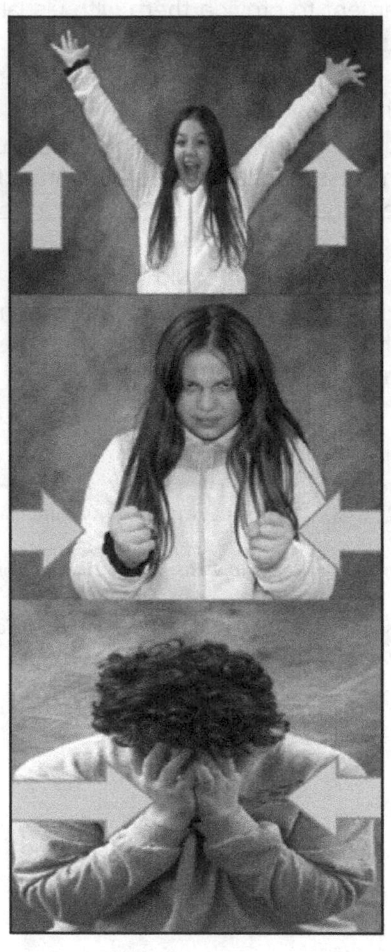

Try it out in the mirror!

You can also show how you are feeling with your posture and legs.

- Upright posture and kick your legs out can show you are excited.
- Raised shoulders and legs closed tightly together can show you are angry.
- Head down forward and legs facing inward can show you are sad.

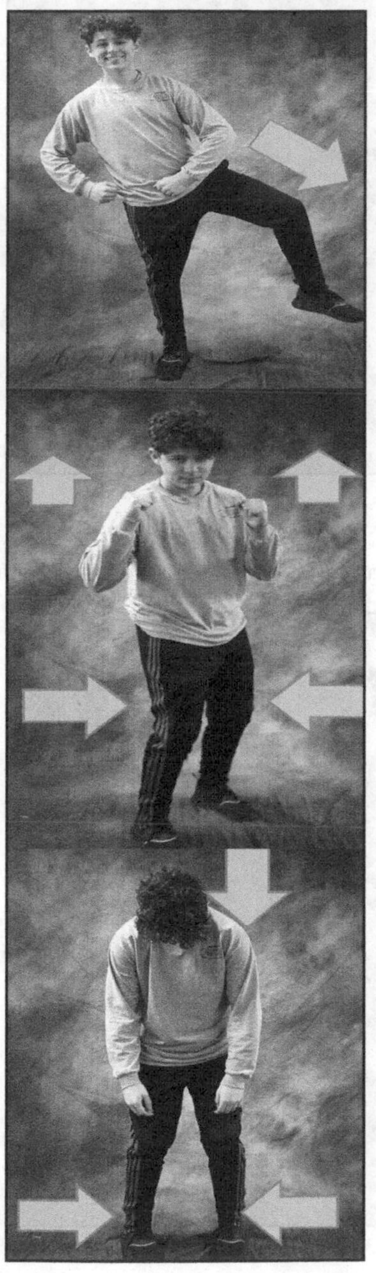

Try it out in the mirror!

A person can also move his or her body to be funny.
You can make big movements with your arms and hands to be funny.

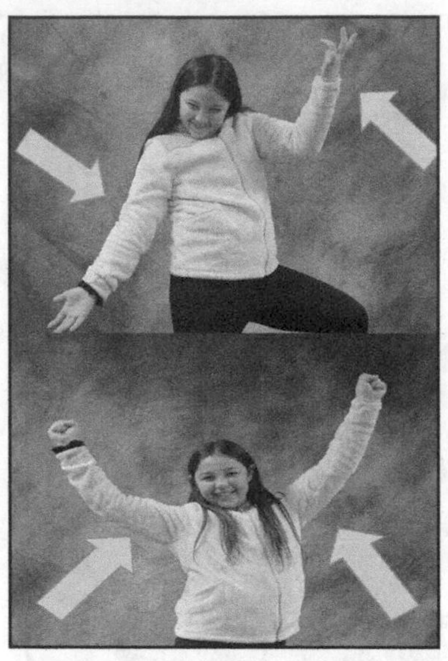

You can make big movements with your legs to be funny.

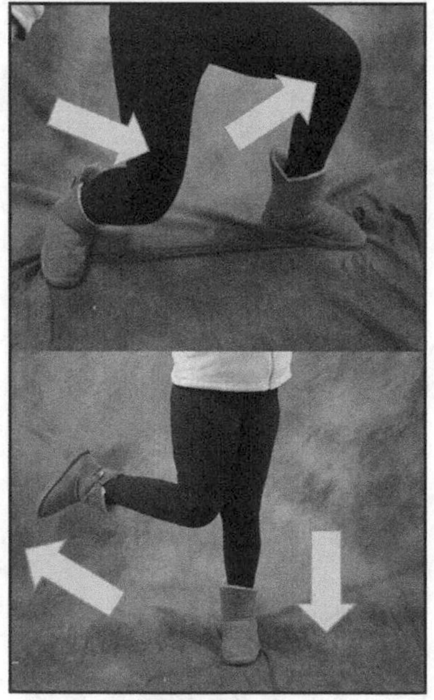

You can wiggle your hands/arms fast or slow to be funny.

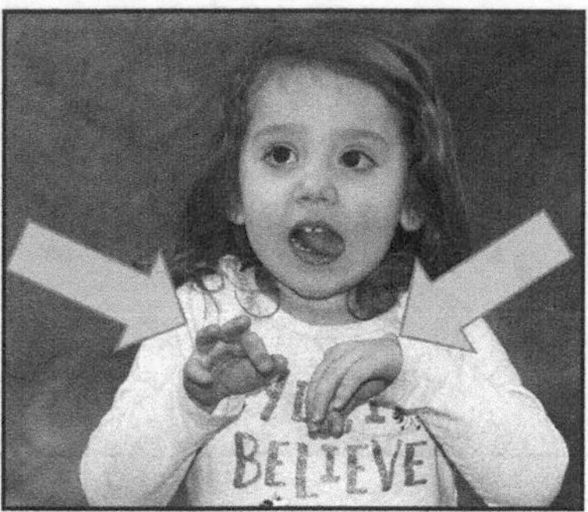

You can make fast or slow movements with your legs to be funny.

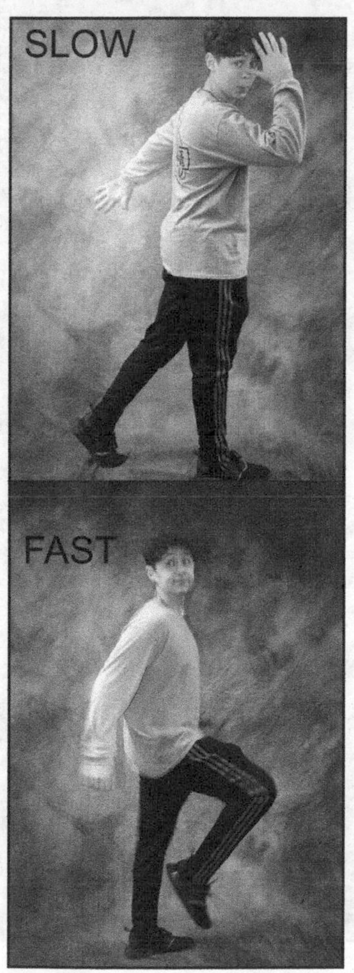

You can also make gestures with your hands to be funny.

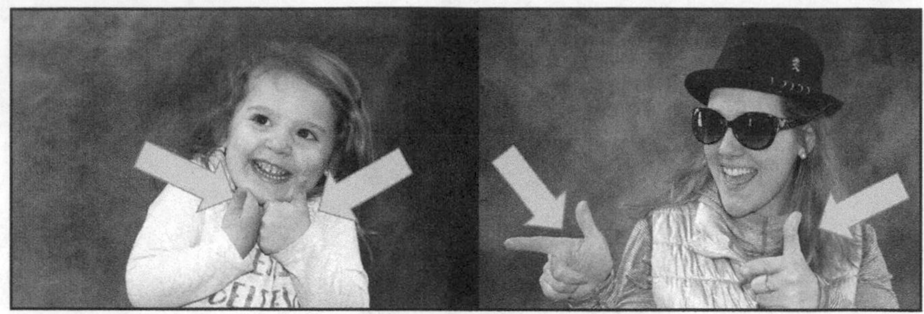

You can move all of your body parts at once to be funny!

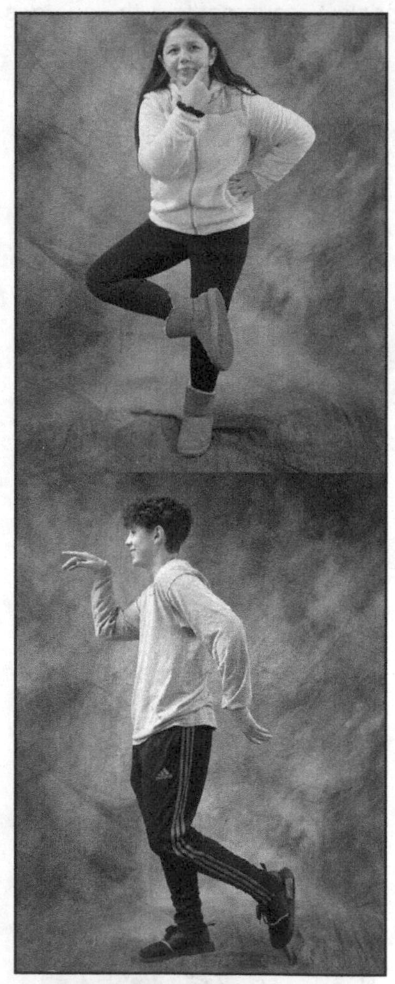

REVIEW QUESTIONS: FUNNY BODY

Name: ______________________________

1. What might a person's arms/hands look like when he or she is sad?
   A. Fingers pointing to sky
   B. Fingers spread out
   C. Hands covering face

2. When a person is angry, he or she might show it by _______.
   A. Raising shoulders
   B. Turning legs inward
   C. Kicking legs out

3. What is the person in the picture feeling?
   A. Excited
   B. Sad
   C. Angry

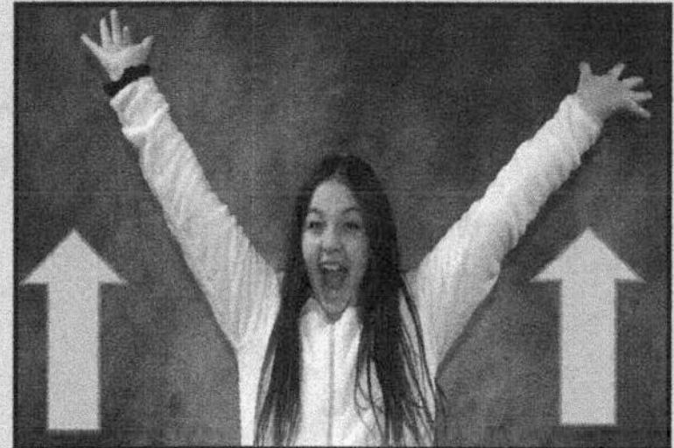

4. What is your favorite funny move? Make it in front of the mirror.

5. You can move your legs __________ to be funny.
   A. Fast
   B. Quietly
   C. Small

Funny Body Review Questions Answer Key

1. C
2. A
3. A
4. No wrong answer
5. A

CHAPTER 4

Physical Comedy

Costumes and Impressions

LESSON 1: FUNNY COSTUMES

Objectives

The participant may:

- Identify the incongruency between funny costumes vs. regular clothes
- Understand how a person can wear costumes to be funny and interact with others

Background

After children have begun to navigate the environment and are able to manipulate objects more skillfully, they begin to retrieve objects and use them to interact with a caregiver (Malik & Marwaha, 2019). In Stage 2 of McGhee's humor development, toddlers also begin to use objects in an unusual or incongruous way because they find it humorous (Semrud-Clikeman & Glass, 2010). Costumes, especially large and colorful ones, are a visually entertaining way to "tickle the funny bone" of a person who is just beginning to develop an awareness of humor, as they are articles of clothing that people do not typically wear (Samson, 2013). This lesson encourages participants to find the humor when one wears funny costumes.

Chaiet, R. *What's So Funny?: Humor-Based Activities for Social Skill Development* (pp. 35-52).

Materials

- Funny Costumes Visual Story
- Review Questions and Answer Key
- Funny hats (two to three minimum)
- Funny wigs (two to three minimum)
- Funny sunglasses/glasses (two to three minimum)
- Funny necklaces, neckties, bows, etc. (two to three minimum)
- Handheld mirror

Preparation

- Use the book or photocopy and staple together the visual story entitled Funny Costumes
- Photocopy Review Questions, one for each participant
- Organize costumes by type into boxes or bags

Procedure

- Read the visual story to the participants or have them take turns reading each page. When there are questions, be sure to engage the participants and allow them to answer using their specific mode of communication (speech, communication device, sign language, gestures, etc.). For participants who seem to have a good basic understanding of the concepts in this lesson, ask more challenging questions that make the material more relatable, such as, "Have you ever worn a funny costume? What was it for? What did it look like?"
- Follow up the activity by having each participant answer the Review Questions, providing assistance as needed. After the participant(s) has completed the questions, the answers given can be compared with the Answer Key.
- Extension activities for this lesson could be:
    - Showing the participants additional photographs of people wearing costumes to be funny (e.g., clowns, individuals wearing Halloween costumes) and asking them what makes the costumes funny

References

Malik, F., & Marwaha, R. (2019). *Developmental stages of social emotional development in children.* StatPearls Publishing.

Samson, A. (2013). Humor(lessness) elucidated—Sense of humor in individuals with autism spectrum disorders: Review and introduction. *Humor, 26*(3), 393-409.

Semrud-Clikeman, M., & Glass, K. (2010). The relation of humor and child development: Social, adaptive and emotional aspects. *Journal of Child Neurology, 25*(10), 1248-1260.

EXERCISE: FUNNY COSTUMES

Something else that you can do to be funny is wear silly costumes. Can you think of who wears costumes to be funny? These people wear costumes to be funny!

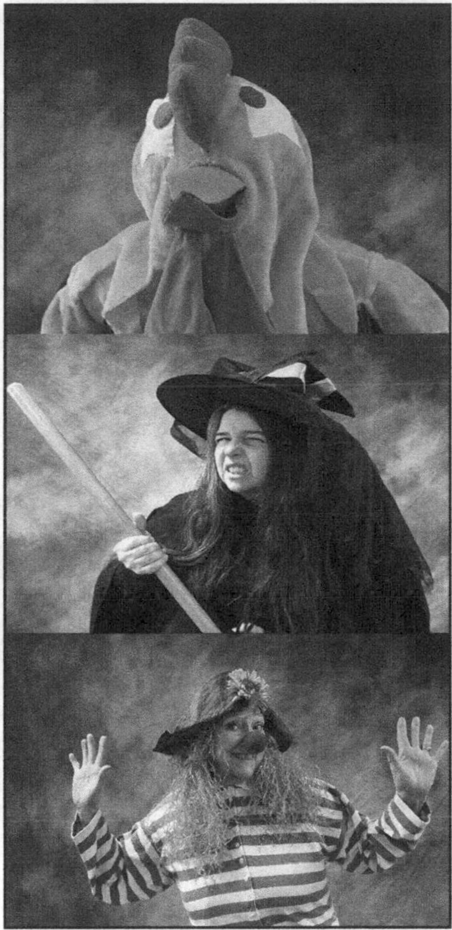

Sports Team Mascots

Halloween Costumes

Clowns

Costumes like this are funny because people do not normally wear things that look like that.

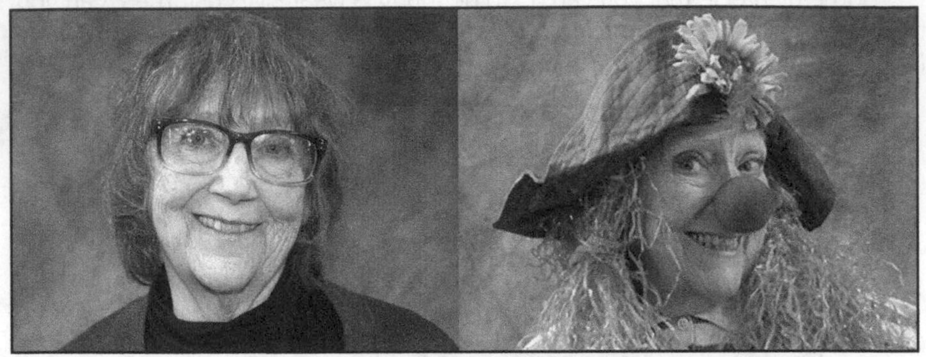

Normal *Costume*

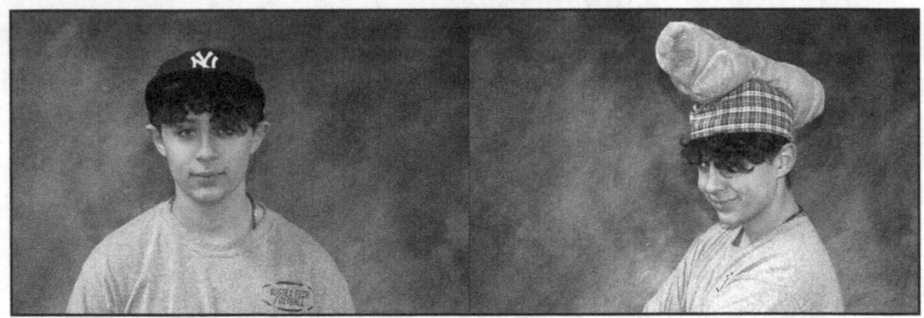

Normal Hat *Funny Hat*

What Is the Difference Between a Normal Hat and a Funny Costume Hat?

- Is it bigger or smaller than normal?
- Does it have a funny shape?
- Does it have crazy patterns?

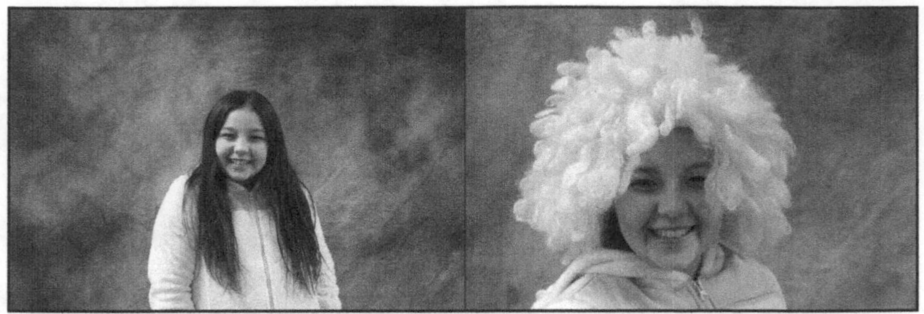

Normal Hair *Funny Hair*

What Is the Difference Between Normal Hair and Funny Hair?

- Is it bigger or smaller than normal?
- Does it have a funny shape?
- Is it a crazy color?

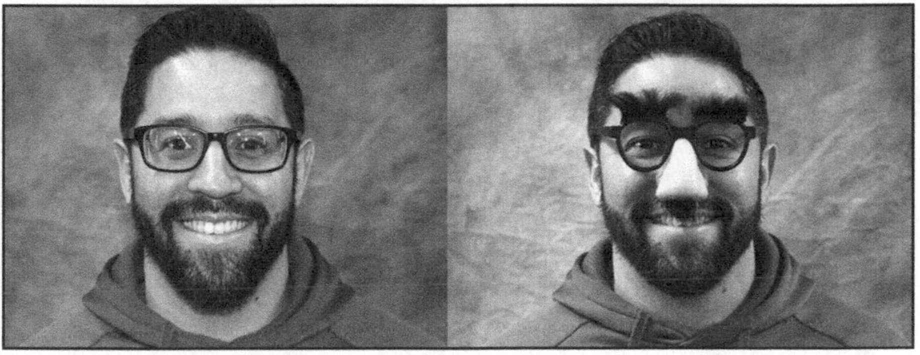

Normal Glasses *Funny Glasses*

What Is the Difference Between Normal Glasses and Funny Glasses?

- Are they bigger or smaller than normal?
- Do they have funny things on them?

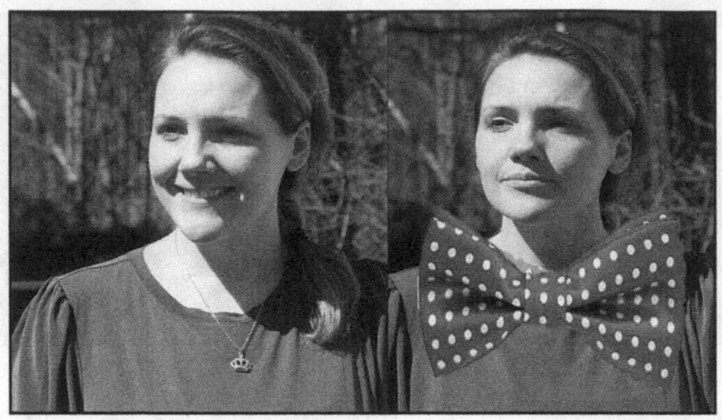

Normal Neckwear *Funny Neckwear*

What Is the Difference Between Normal Neckwear and Funny Neckwear?

- Is it bigger or smaller than normal?
- Does it have funny things on it?

ACTIVITIES: FUNNY COSTUMES

Let's try some funny hats!

1. Take a hat.
2. Put it on and look in the mirror.
3. Do you look funny?
   Yes No
4. What makes the hat funny?
   Size? Shape? Silly decoration? Color?
5. Pass the hat to a friend/the instructor.
6. Does he or she look funny?
   Yes No

Let's try some wigs!

1. Take a wig.
2. Put it on and look in the mirror.
3. Do you look funny?
   Yes No
4. What makes the wig funny?
   Size? Shape? Silly decoration? Color?
5. Pass it to a friend/the instructor.
6. Does he or she look funny?
   Yes No

Let's try some glasses!

1. Take a pair of glasses.
2. Put them on and look in the mirror.
3. Do you look funny?
   Yes No
4. What makes the glasses funny?
   Size? Shape? Silly decoration? Color?
5. Pass them on to a friend/the instructor.
6. Does he or she look funny?
   Yes No

Let's try some neckwear!

1. Take a piece of neckwear.
2. Put it on and look in the mirror.
3. Do you look funny?
   Yes No
4. What makes the neckwear funny?
   Size? Shape? Silly decoration? Color?
5. Pass it on to a friend/the instructor.
6. Does he or she look funny?
   Yes No

Put together a crazy outfit!

1. Each person takes a piece of neckwear, a wig, a hat, and a pair of glasses.
2. Put them all on at one time and look in the mirror.
3. Do you look funny?
   Yes No
4. Does your friend/the instructor look funny?
   Yes No
5. Who looks the funniest?

REVIEW QUESTIONS: FUNNY COSTUMES

Name: ______________________________

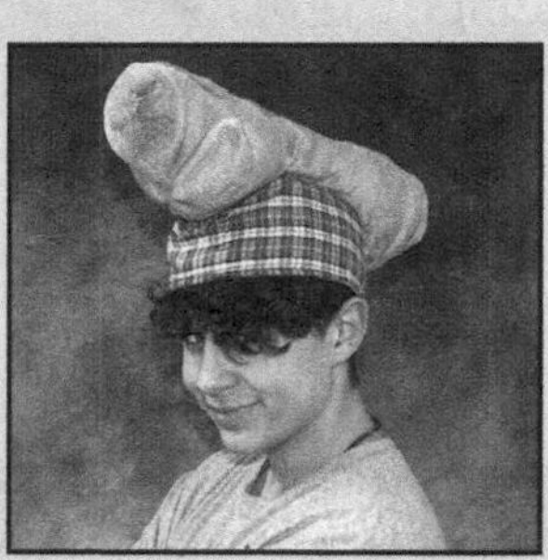

1. What costume is this person wearing to be funny?
   A. Funny hat
   B. Funny wig
   C. Funny neckwear

2. Why is the costume in Question 1 funny?
   A. Very small
   B. Funny color
   C. Funny shape

3. Who wears costumes to be funny?
   A. Teacher
   B. Clown
   C. Mailman

4. Which glasses are funny?

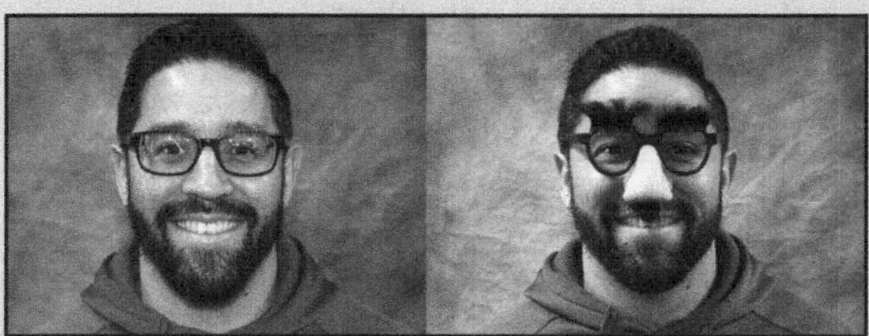

A. B.

5. Why are the glasses in Question 4 funny?
   A. Very big
   B. Funny color
   C. Funny things on them

Funny Costumes Review Questions Answer Key

1. A
2. C
3. B
4. B
5. C

Lesson 2: Impressions

Objectives

The participant may:

- Increase awareness of different facial expressions
- Increase awareness of different types of body language
- Understand how a person can use basic impressions to be funny and interact with others

Background

In the next phase of social-emotional development, toddlers typically begin to engage in pretend play (Malik & Marwaha, 2019). They do this by imitating the emotions, body language, and speech/sounds of people and animals they observe in their environment. Doing basic impressions of familiar characters allows the participants to practice pretend play in a more structured way. Impressions may be funny to participants because they involve incongruity of facial expressions and body language, as people do not typically act like the characters being imitated. This lesson encourages participants to do impressions of familiar characters in order to be funny and interact with others.

Materials

- Impressions Visual Story
- Review Questions and Answer Key
- Full-length mirror
- Costume pieces for princess, zombie, cowboy, and super hero (optional)

Preparation

- Use the book or photocopy and staple together the visual story entitled Impressions
- Photocopy Review Questions, one for each participant

Procedure

- Read the visual story to the participants or have them take turns reading each page. When there are questions, be sure to engage the participants and allow them to answer using their specific mode of communication (speech, communication device, sign language, gestures, etc.).
- When introducing each impression, first show them by modeling it. Be sure to use exaggerated movements and facial expressions.
- Encourage participants to look in the mirror each time they are asked to do an impression to provide them with visual feedback of the body language and expressions they are using.
- If doing this activity with a group, encourage participants to look at the body movements and facial expressions of their peers.
- Follow up the activity by having each participant answer the Review Questions, providing assistance as needed. After the participant(s) has completed the questions, the answers given can be compared with the Answer Key.
- Extension activities for this lesson could be:
    - Showing the participants video clips of comedians who do impressions or doing additional impressions of familiar commercial characters

Reference

Malik, F., & Marwaha, R. (2019). *Developmental stages of social emotional development in children.* StatPearls Publishing.

EXERCISE: IMPRESSIONS

Today, we are going to do impressions and use our face, body, and voice to be funny. Impressions are when you act like another person. When you do an impression of someone, you want to make the same faces that person makes.

You want to make your eyes and eyebrows do the same thing that theirs do.

- Point to your eyebrows
- Look at your eyebrows in the mirror
- Point to your eyes
- Look at your eyes in the mirror

What do their eyes and eyebrows look like? Try making those movements with your eyes and eyebrows while looking in a mirror.

How do their eyes and eyebrows look?

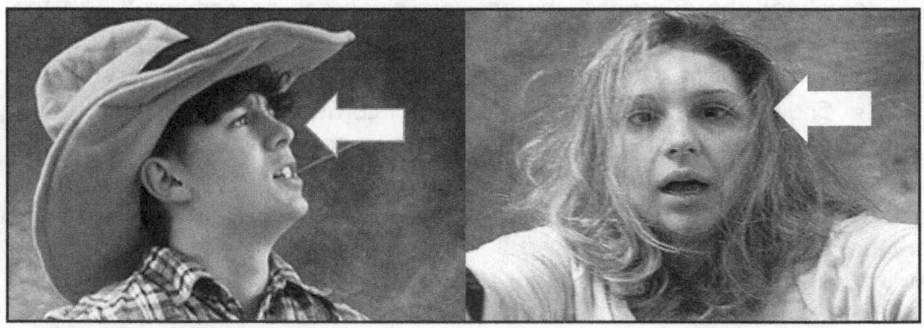

Cowboy

- Squinting eyes
- Scrunched eyebrows

Zombie

- Wide staring eyes
- Eyebrows stay still

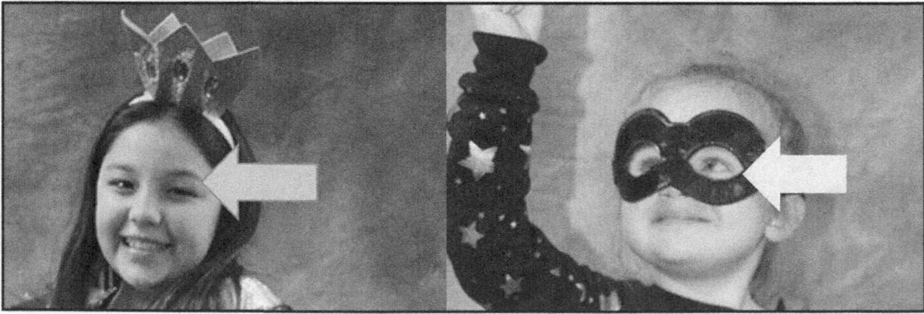

Princess

- Batting eyelashes
- Eyebrows raised

Superhero

- Wide open eyes, looking up

You want to make your mouth do the same thing that theirs does.

- Point to your mouth
- Look at your mouth in the mirror

What do their mouths look like? Try making those movements with your mouth while looking in a mirror.

How do their mouths look?

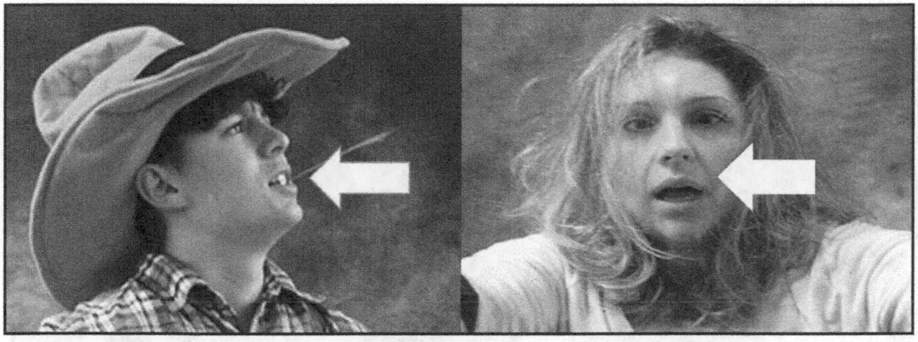

Cowboy *Zombie*

- Teeth clenched
- Open wide

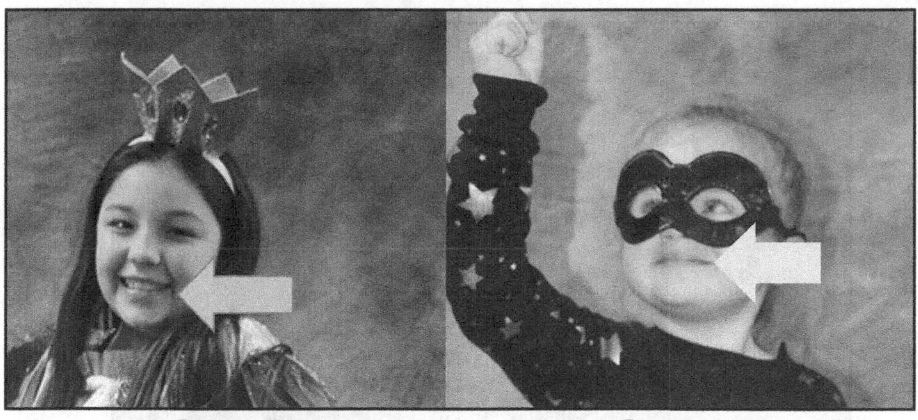

Princess *Superhero*

- Smiling
- Smiling

When you do an impression, you also want to try to make your arms do the same thing as theirs do.

- Point to your arms
- Look at your arms in the mirror

What do their arms look like? Try making those movements with your arms while looking in a mirror.

How do their arms look?

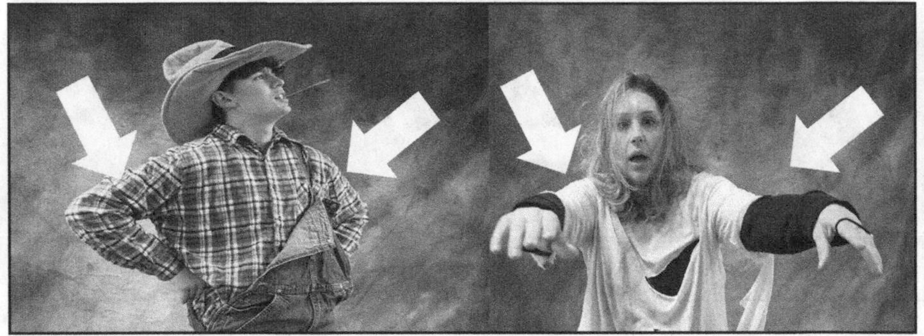

Cowboy

- Hands on hips

Zombie

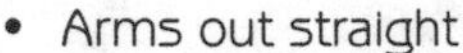

- Arms out straight

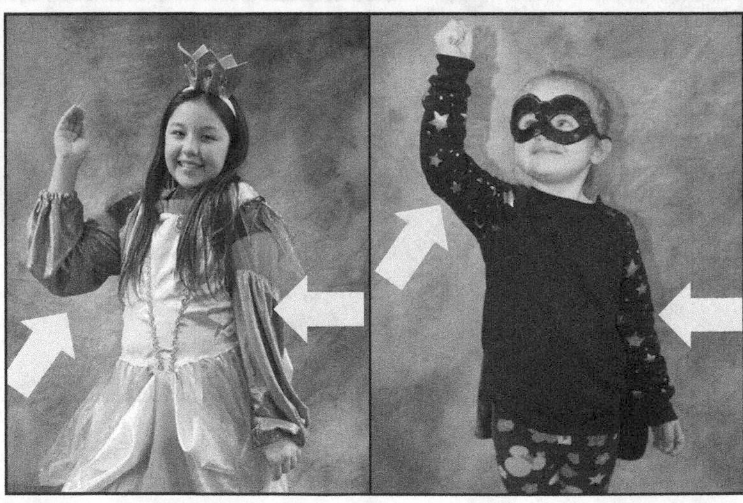

Princess

- One arm doing a princess wave
- Other hand holding her dress

Superhero

- One arm up, hand in a fist
- Other arm down

What voice does that person use? What does he or she say? Try saying it the same way the person would.

How does his or her voice sound? What does he or she say?

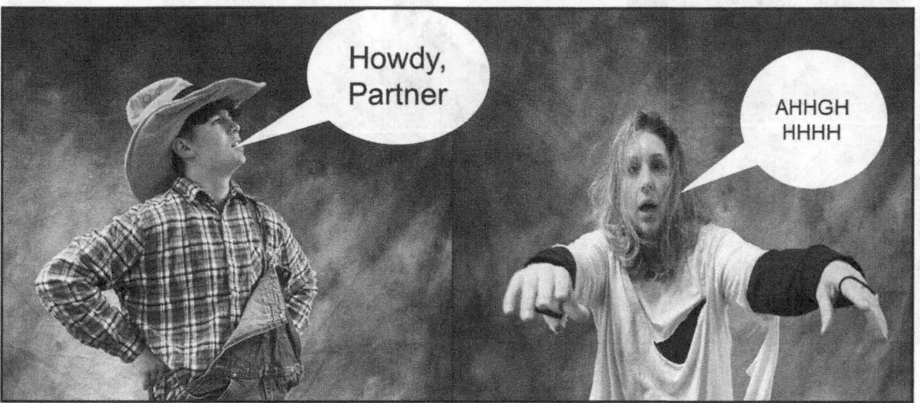

Cowboy

- Low, raspy voice
- "Howdy, partner"

Zombie

- Low, scary voice
- "AHHGHHHHH"

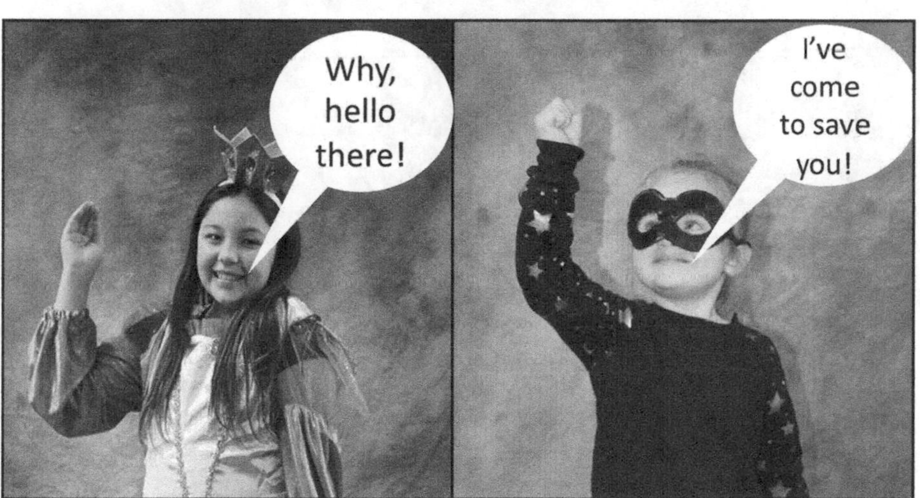

Princess

- High, sweet voice
- "Why, hello there!"

Superhero

- Low, confident voice
- "I've come to save you!"

Let's put it all together and practice our impressions!

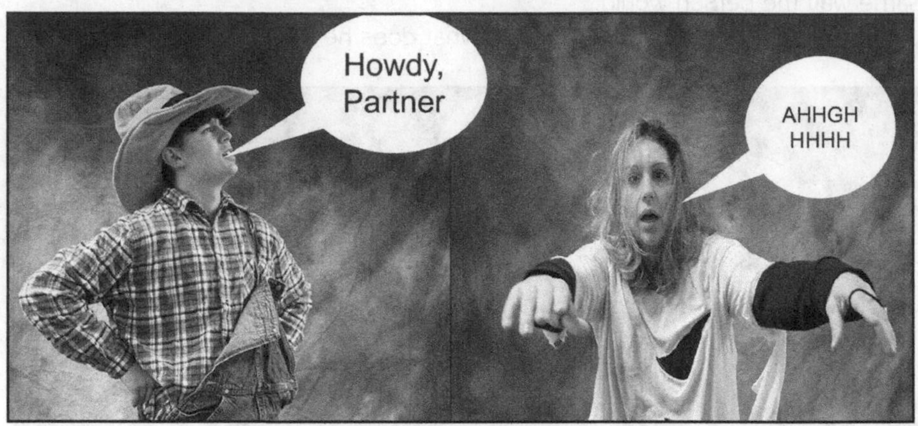

Cowboy

- Squinting eyes
- Scrunched eyebrows
- Teeth clenched
- Hands on hips
- "Howdy, partner"

Zombie

- Wide staring eyes
- Eyebrows still
- Mouth open wide
- Arms out straight
- "AHHGHHHHH"

Let's put it all together and practice our impressions!

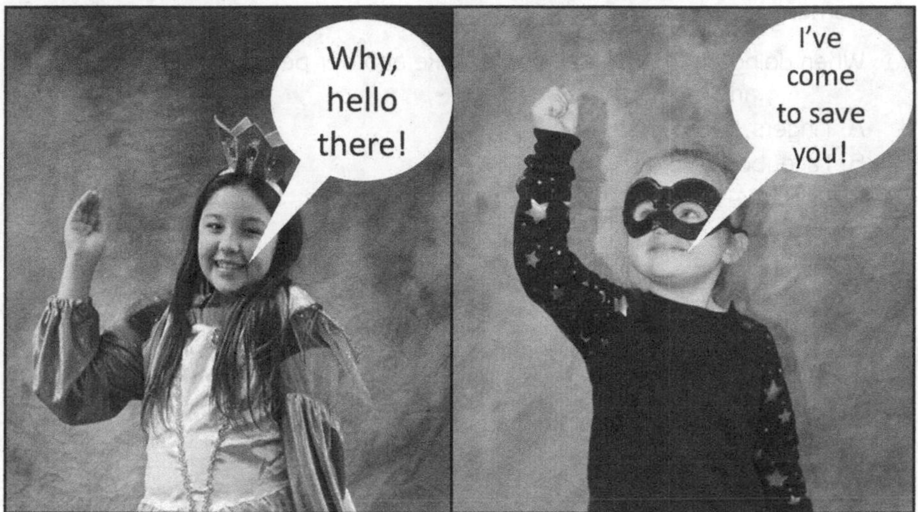

Princess	*Superhero*
• Batting eyelashes • Eyebrows raised • Smiling • One arm doing a princess wave • Other hand holding dress • "Why, hello there!"	• Wide-open eyes, looking up • Smiling • One arm up, hand in a fist • Other arm down • "I've come to save you!"

REVIEW QUESTIONS: IMPRESSIONS

Name: ______________________________

1. When doing an impression, you act like another person using your _____, _______, and ______.
   A. Fingers, toes, knees
   B. Face, body, voice
   C. Ears, eyes, nose

2. When you do an impression of a zombie, you should make your eyes:
   A. Wide and staring
   B. Squinted
   C. Eyelashes batting

3. When you do an impression of a princess, you could say:
   A. "Howdy, partner"
   B. "AHHGHHHHH"
   C. "Why, hello there!"

4. When you do an impression of a cowboy, you put your arms:
   A. Straight out
   B. On your hips
   C. Folded together

5. What was your favorite impression today? Do that impression while looking in the mirror.

Impressions Review Questions Answer Key

1. B
2. A
3. C
4. B
5. No wrong answer

CHAPTER 5

Physical Comedy

Slapstick

Lesson 1: Introduction to Slapstick

Objectives

The participant may:

- Continue to increase awareness of facial expressions and body language
- Understand the difference between slapstick and someone getting injured
- Understand how a person can use exaggerated facial expressions and body movements with slapstick to be funny and interact with peers

Background

As creativity and imagination continue to develop, a child's pretend play scenarios eventually become more complex (Malik & Marwaha, 2019). They begin to enjoy humor that is a little more involved as well, yet still physical and visual in nature. Slapstick uses big facial expressions and movements, but also incorporates incongruous scenarios, such as slipping on a banana peel or running into a wall. While children often begin to enjoy slapstick around 2 years of age, it continues to be enjoyable up through middle childhood, until a developmental age of approximately 11 years (Buijzen & Valkenburg, 2004). In addition, studies have shown that slapstick is the only type of humor that is appreciated by children with autism spectrum disorder and other intellectual disabilities as much as same-aged peers (Agius & Levey, 2019). This lesson introduces slapstick and encourages participants to act out silly scenarios in order to be funny and interact with others.

Chaiet, R. *What's So Funny?: Humor-Based Activities for Social Skill Development* (pp. 53-78).

Materials

- Slapstick Visual Story
- Review Questions and Answer Key
- Small, empty cardboard box
- Printed image of banana

Preparation

- Use the book or photocopy and staple together the visual story entitled Slapstick
- Photocopy Review Questions, one for each participant
- Copy and cut out image of a banana and laminate, if possible
- Clear an area in the room for participants to make big movements
- A clear wall that is free of hangings should be available to do the Running Into a Wall activity

Procedure

- Read the visual story to the participants or have them take turns reading each page. When there are questions, be sure to engage the participants and allow them to answer using their specific mode of communication (speech, communication device, sign language, gestures, etc.). For participants who seem to have a good basic understanding of the concepts in this lesson, ask more challenging questions that make the material more relatable, such as, "Have you ever seen a character in a movie or cartoon pretend to get injured in a funny way? What are some examples?"
- When introducing each slapstick activity, first show them by modeling the activity. Be sure to use exaggerated facial expressions and movements.
- Follow up the activity by having each participant answer the Review Questions, providing assistance as needed. After the participant(s) has completed the questions, the answers given can be compared with the Answer Key.
- Extension activities for this lesson could be:
    - Showing the participants video clips of slapstick, either in its original form (e.g., Charlie Chaplin, *The Three Stooges*) or how it is often featured today in cartoons (e.g., *Looney Tunes*, *Spongebob Squarepants*)

References

Agius, J., & Levey, S. (2019). Humor intervention approaches for children, adolescents and adults. *Israeli Journal for Humor Research, 8*(1), 8-28.

Buijzen, M., & Valkenburg, P. (2004). Developing a typology of humor in audiovisual media. *Media Psychology, 6*, 147-167.

Malik, F., & Marwaha, R. (2019). *Developmental stages of social emotional development in children.* StatPearls Publishing.

EXERCISE: SLAPSTICK

Today, we are going to talk about slapstick. Slapstick is when people act out a clumsy or embarrassing situation to be funny. In slapstick, people might pretend to fall down or run into things that may hurt you if it was real, but in slapstick, it is pretend and is just to be funny. Let's look at the difference between slapstick and when a person does get hurt.

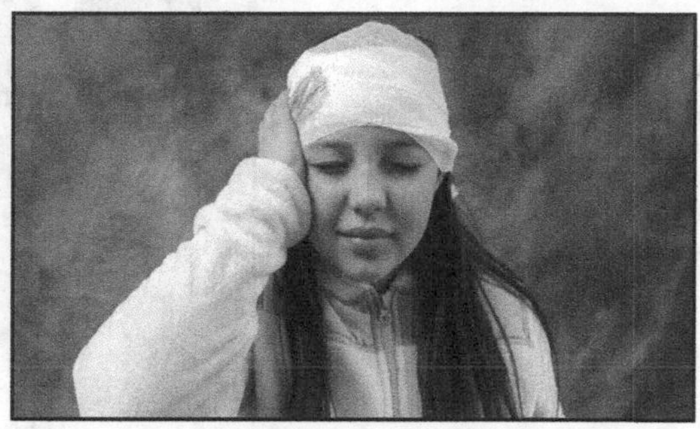

The Person Is Really Hurt

- He or she is crying
- He or she is bleeding or injured
- NOT FUNNY

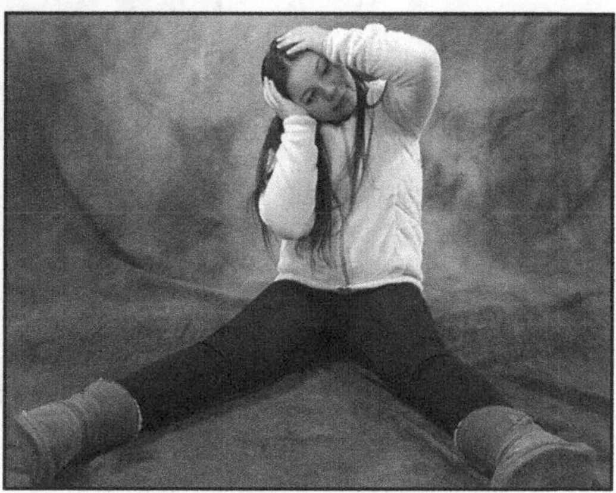

The Person Is Doing Slapstick

- He or she is making a silly expression
- He or she is not really hurt or bleeding
- FUNNY

When you do slapstick, you can use the same funny big arms/legs and funny faces we talked about before to act out the clumsy situation.

ACTIVITIES: SLAPSTICK

First, we are going to try "Dropping a Box"

You are going to use big, silly faces and body movements while you first pretend to pick up a heavy box and then pretend to drop it on your toe!

What Does Your Face and Body Do When You Carry Something Heavy in Slapstick?

- Eyebrows down
- Teeth grimacing
- Arms holding object wide
- Legs spread wide
- Say: "UHHHHH!"

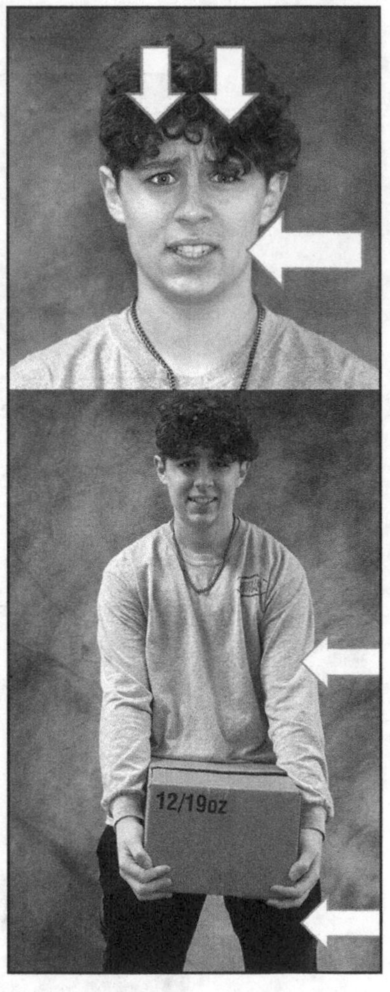

What Does Your Face and Body Do When You Drop Something on Your Toe in Slapstick?

- Eyebrows up
- Mouth open
- Holding one foot
- Jumping up and down
- Say: "OWWWW!"

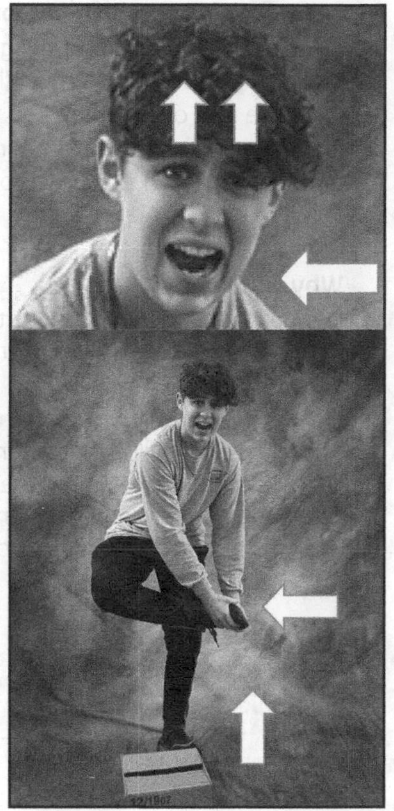

Let's Act Out "Dropping a Box"

- Make a strained face and struggle to pick up a box as you say "UHHHHH!"
- Drop the box on your toe
- Make an ouch face, hold your foot, and jump up and down as you say "OWWWW!"

Why Is It Funny?

- Did someone REALLY get hurt? No! If he or she were really injured, it would not be funny.
- Do people usually make big faces and movements like that when they drop something on their toe? No! The funny faces and movements are what makes it funny to look at!

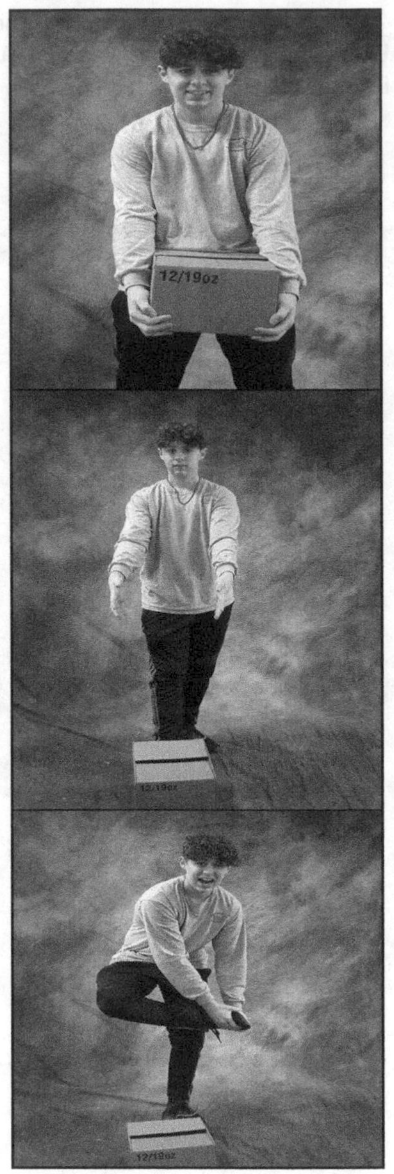

Next, we will try "Running Into a Wall"

You are going to use big, silly faces and body movements to pretend to run into a wall and then slide down it slowly like a cartoon!

What Does Your Face and Body Do When You Are Running in Slapstick?

- Eyebrows down
- Blow air through lips
- Move arms up and down with elbows bent
- High knees up and down

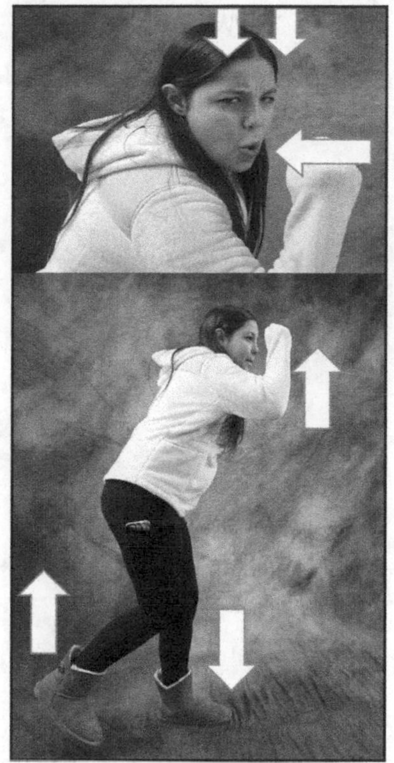

What Does Your Face and Body Do When You Run Into a Wall in Slapstick?

- Run into wall and freeze
- Slide whole body down the wall slowly
- Say: "OWWWW!"

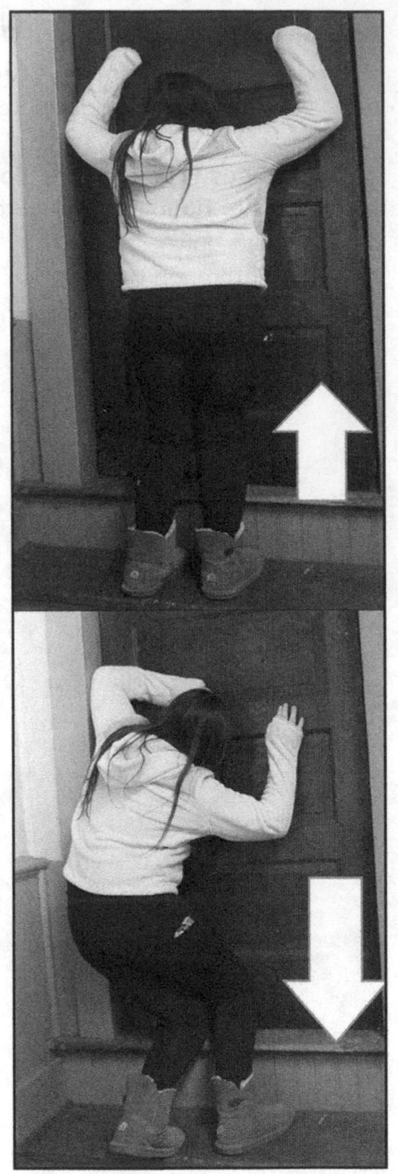

Let's Act Out "Running Into a Wall"

- Pretend to run slowly
- When you reach the wall, pretend to hit it and then freeze
- Say "OWWWW!" as you slowly slide body down the wall

Why Is It Funny?

- Did someone REALLY get hurt? No! If he or she were really injured, it would not be funny.
- Do people usually run into walls and slide down them like that? No! It is funny to see a person run into and slide down a wall like he or she is a cartoon!

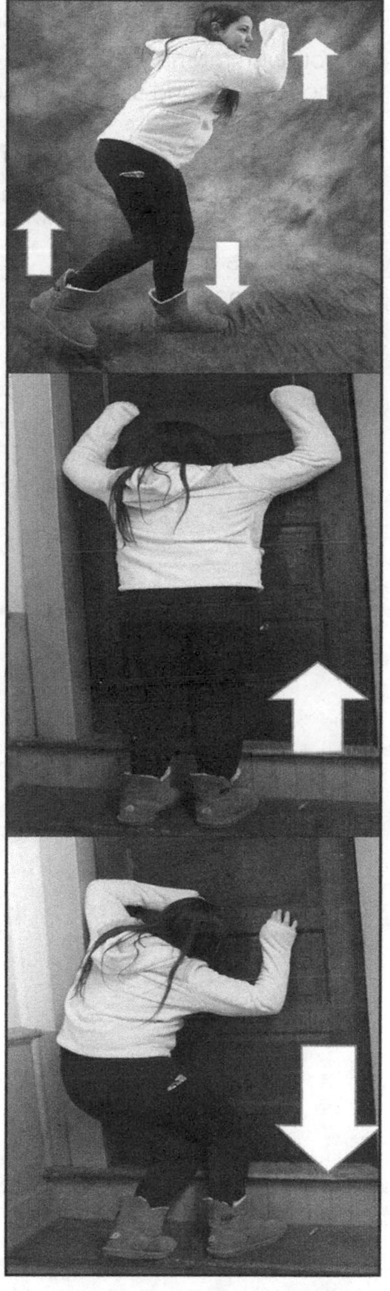

Last, we will try "Slipping on a Banana Peel"

You will pretend to step on a banana peel, slip on it, and make big arm and leg movements and silly faces like you are slipping!

What Does Your Face and Body Do When You Slip on Something in Slapstick?

- Eyebrows up
- Mouth open, scared
- Wave arms up and down fast
- Legs move up and down fast
- Say: "WHOOAA!"

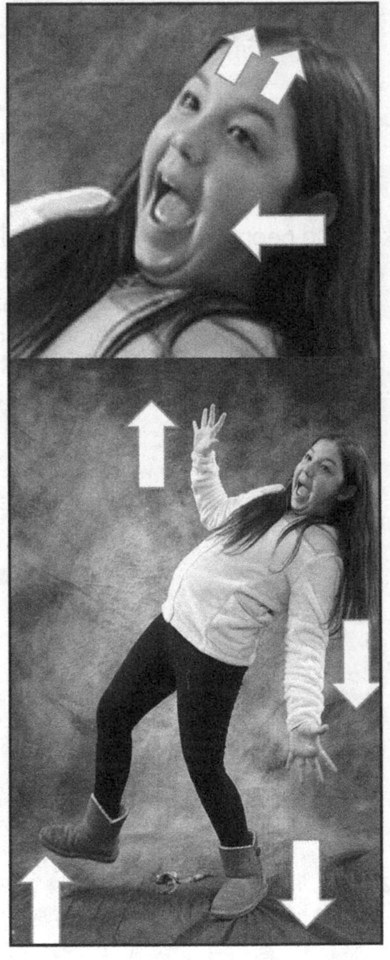

Let's Act Out "Slipping on a Banana Peel"

- Walk toward the banana peel and then step on it
- Make big leg and arm movements like you are slipping
- Make a scared face as you say "WHOOAA!"

Why Is It Funny?

- Did the person REALLY get hurt? No! If he or she were really injured, it would not be funny.
- Do people really slip on banana peels? No! It is funny to think of someone slipping on a banana peel like a cartoon.
- Do people really make big faces and movements like that when they slip on something? No! The funny faces and movements are what makes it funny to look at!

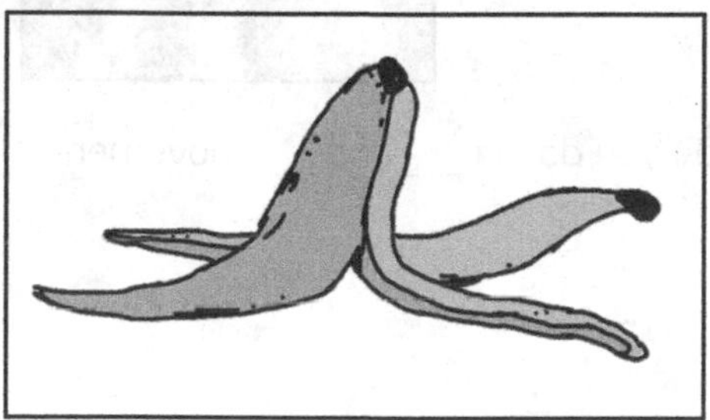

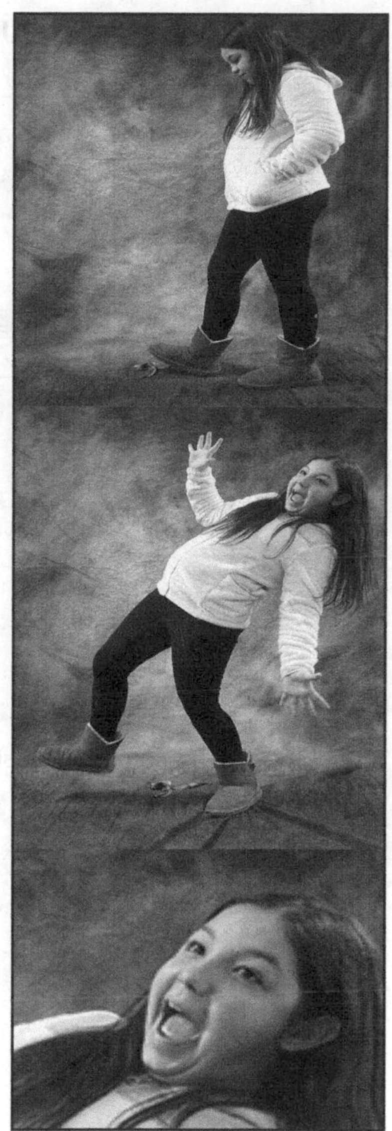

REVIEW QUESTIONS: SLAPSTICK

Name:______________________________

1. __________ is when people act out a clumsy or embarrassing situation to be funny.
   A. Chopstick
   B. Slapchop
   C. Slapstick

2. In slapstick, people may pretend to slip, drop something on themselves, or run into a wall, but they ______ get hurt.
   A. Do NOT
   B. Definitely
   C. Should

3. Is this person hurt or doing slapstick?
   A. Hurt
   B. Doing slapstick

4. Is this person hurt or doing slapstick?
   A. Hurt
   B. Doing slapstick

5. When you pretend to slip in slapstick, you do big ___ and ___ movements.
   A. Nose, ear
   B. Arm, leg
   C. Hair, toe

Slapstick Review Questions

Answer Key

1. C
2. A
3. B
4. A
5. B

Lesson 2: Messy Slapstick

Objectives

The participant may:

- Continue to increase awareness of facial expressions and body language
- Understand the difference between using messy slapstick to be funny and making big messes in real life
- Understand how a person can use exaggerated facial expressions and body movements with messy slapstick to be funny and interact with others
- Engage in parallel and cooperative play interactions

Background

By the developmental age of 3 years, children begin to participate in more symbolic, pretend play, using objects to represent something they have seen used by adults in real life (Malik & Marwaha, 2019). They begin to interact more with their peers, first engaging in parallel play activities followed by those that require cooperation and turn taking. In this slapstick lesson, basic materials are used by participants to represent different types of food to make the pretend messes. This slapstick lesson continues to use incongruous scenarios, as well as exaggerated expressions and movements, but it requires more complex social interactions than the introductory lesson. The first activity has the individual participate alongside a peer or the instructor, while the second and third activities require a playful, dyadic interaction.

Materials

- Messy Slapstick Visual Story
- Review Questions and Answer Key
- Small bucket
- 25 to 50 colorful craft pompoms or balls made out of colorful craft dough to make "gumballs"
- Food tray
- Three small plastic/paper plates
- Two to four pieces of pretend plastic food
- Two chairs
- Small table or tray
- Yellow yarn or decorative ribbon cut up into small pieces to look like spaghetti

Preparation

- Use the book or photocopy and staple together the visual story entitled Messy Slapstick
- Photocopy Review Questions, one for each participant
- Fill a small bucket with colorful craft pompoms/dough balls
- Put the fake pieces of food on one plastic/paper plate
- Put the plate with the fake food on it on a food tray
- Put the yellow yarn/ribbon on two other small plastic/paper plates
- Clear an area in the room for participants to make big movements and make "pretend messes"

Procedure

- Read the visual story to the participants or have them take turns reading each page. When there are questions, be sure to engage the participants and allow them to answer using their specific mode of communication (speech, communication device, sign language, gestures, etc.). For participants who seem to have a good basic understanding of the concepts in this lesson, ask more challenging questions that make the material more relatable, such as, "Have you ever seen a character in a movie or cartoon make a big mess? What are some examples?"
- When introducing each slapstick activity, first show them by modeling the activity. Be sure to use exaggerated facial expressions and movements.
- Follow up the activity by having each participant answer the Review Questions, providing assistance as needed. After the participant(s) has completed the questions, the answers given can be compared with the Answer Key.
- Extension activities for this lesson could be:
    - Showing the participants video clips of messy slapstick, either in its original form (e.g., Charlie Chaplin, *The Three Stooges*) or how it is often featured today in cartoons (e.g., *Looney Tunes*, *Spongebob Squarepants*)

Reference

Malik, F., & Marwaha, R. (2019). *Developmental stages of social emotional development in children.* StatPearls Publishing.

EXERCISE: MESSY SLAPSTICK

Today, we are going to talk about "messy" slapstick. In messy slapstick, a person will pretend to drop and scatter things or do something else that makes a mess. If it happened in real life, this may make a person feel mad or frustrated, but in slapstick, it is just pretend and is just to be funny! Let's look at the difference between slapstick and when a person makes a real mess.

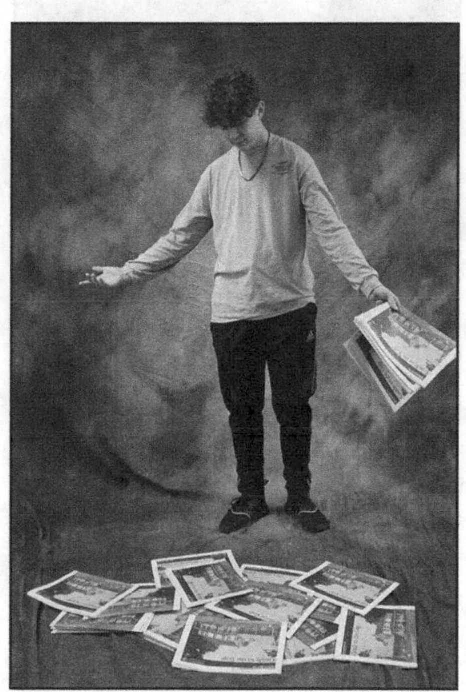

Real Mess

- There is a big mess that is hard to clean
- The person looks really mad or frustrated
- NOT FUNNY

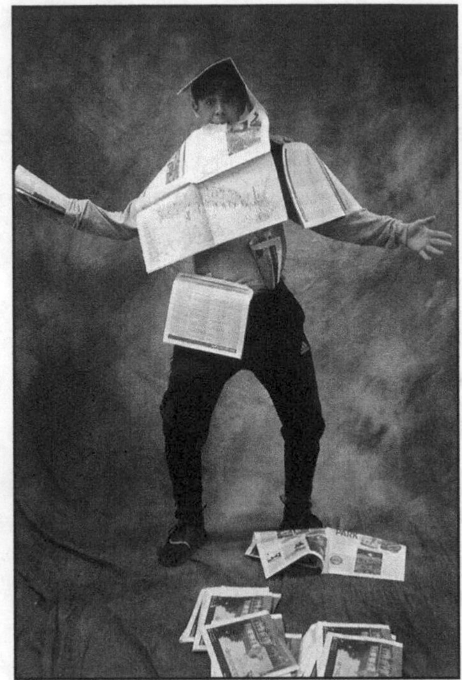

The Person Is Doing Messy Slapstick

- The person is making a silly expression
- The person is using big arm/leg movements
- Not a real mess
- FUNNY

ACTIVITIES: MESSY SLAPSTICK

Let's try some messy slapstick! First, we are going to try "Dropping Gumballs"

- One person will use big, silly faces and body movements and pretend to drop a bunch of gumballs all over the floor!
- Another person will use big, silly faces and body movements and pretend to slip on the gumballs!

What Does Your Face and Body Do When You Make a Mess in Slapstick?

- Eyebrows down
- Nervous teeth grimace
- Hands to side of face
- Legs together
- Say: "OOOPS!"

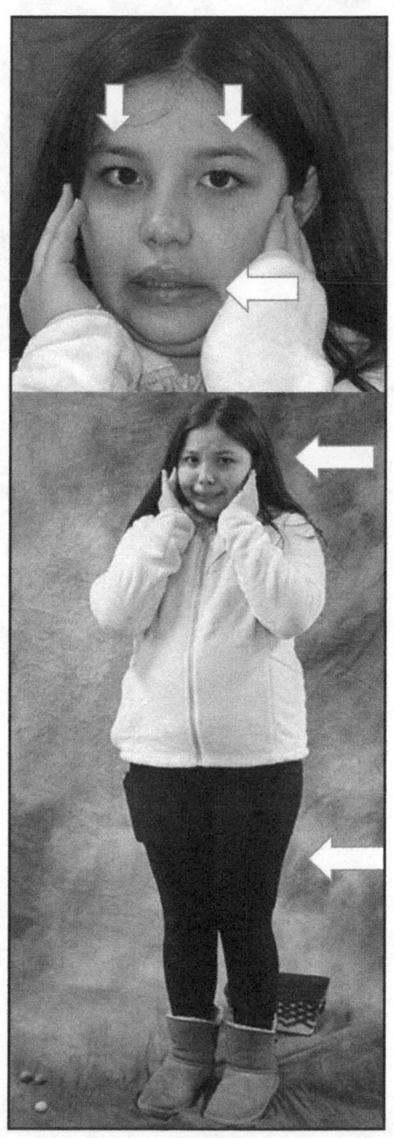

What Does Your Face and Body Do When You Slip on Something in Slapstick?

- Eyebrows up
- Mouth open, scared
- Wave arms up and down fast
- Legs move up and down fast
- Say: "WHOOAA!"

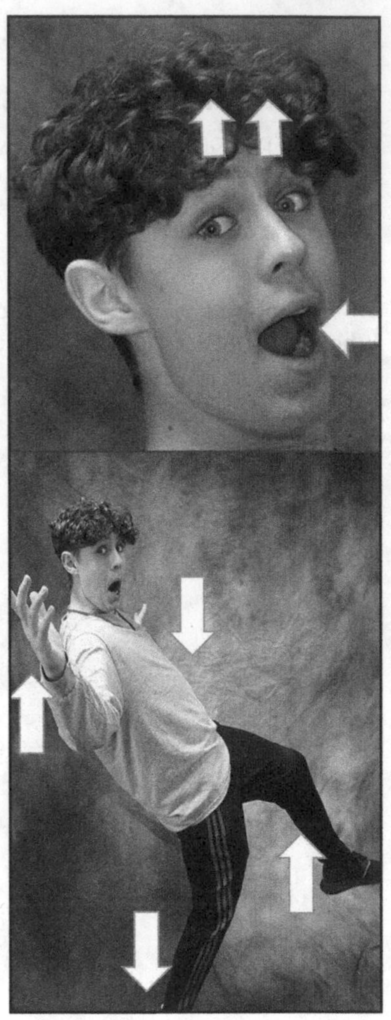

Let's Act Out "Dropping Gumballs"

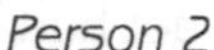

Person 1

- Carry a bucket of colorful pom poms/dough that looks like gumballs
- Pretend to trip and throw gumballs in the air
- Say "OOOPS!" with nervous face

Person 2

- Walk onto the gumballs
- Pretend to slip on them by making big leg and arm movements
- Say "WHOOAA!" with scared face

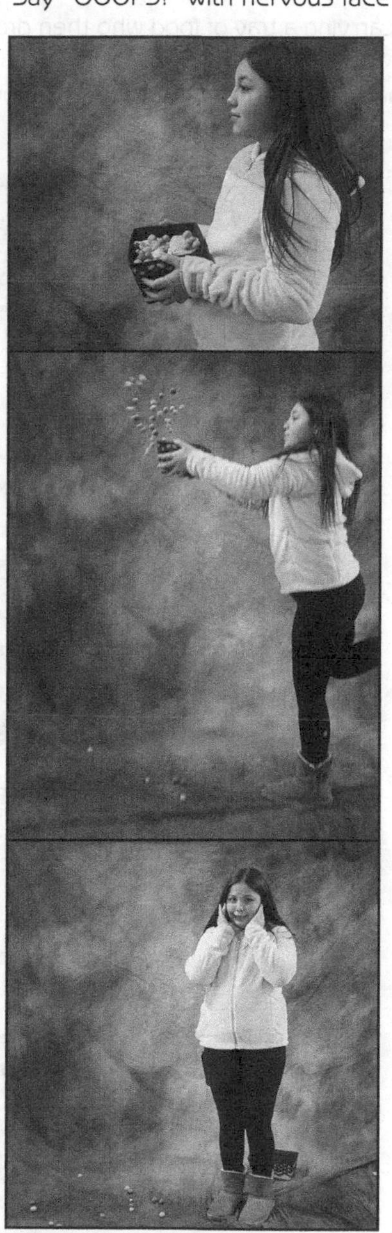

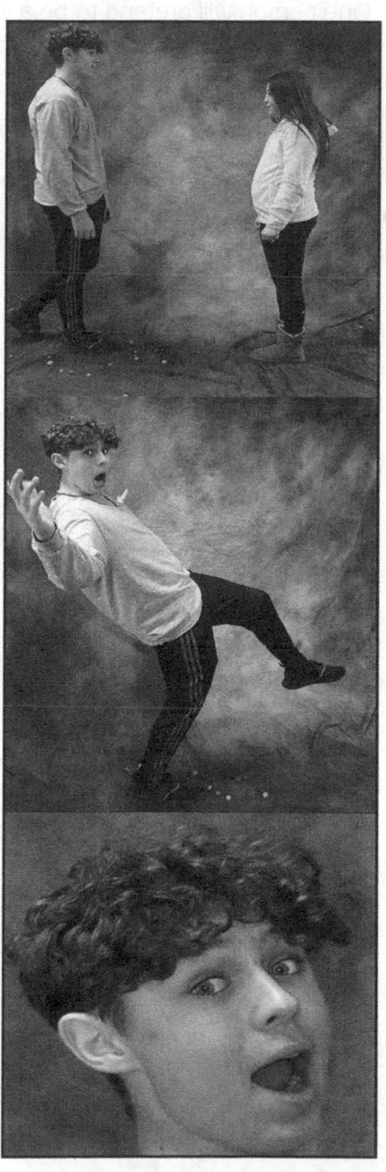

Why Is It Funny?

- Did someone REALLY get hurt? No! If he or she were really injured, it would not be funny.
- Do people really act like this when they slip? No! The funny faces and big movements are what makes it funny to look at!

Next, we will try "Dropping the Food Order"

- One person will pretend to be a waiter carrying a tray of food who then drops the food on the customer
- Another person pretends to be the unhappy customer whose food is all over him or her

What Does Your Face and Body Do When You Make a Mess?

- Eyebrows down
- Nervous teeth grimace
- Shrugging shoulders
- Say: "OOOPS!"

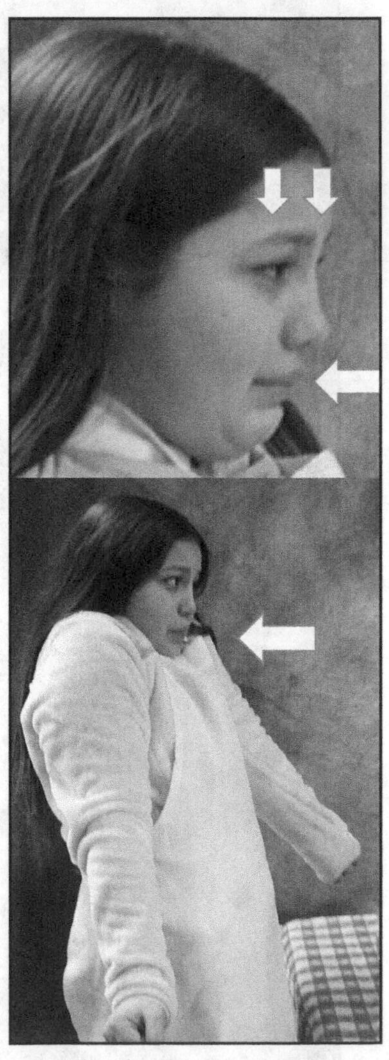

What Does Your Face and Body Do When Something Spills on You in Slapstick?

- Eyebrows down
- Mouth closed, angry
- Shake finger at the waiter
- Say: "GRRRRRR!"

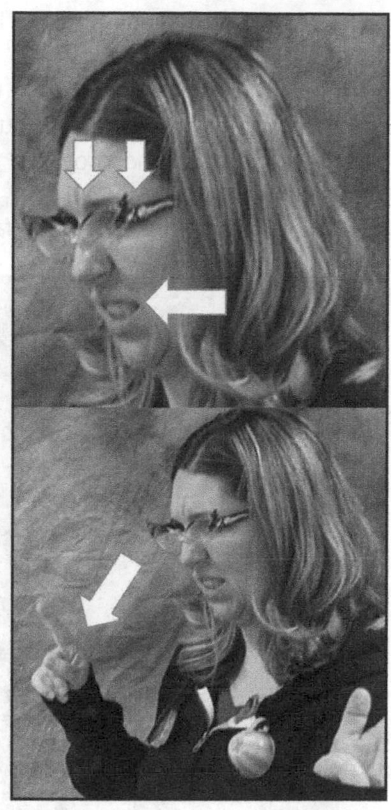

Let's Act Out "Dropping the Food Order"

Person 1

- Carry a tray of pretend food over to the other person who is sitting
- Pretend to trip and drop the food on the person
- Say "OOOPS!" with nervous face

Person 2 (seated)

- Make a pretend angry face
- Shake your finger at the waiter
- Say "GRRRRRR!"

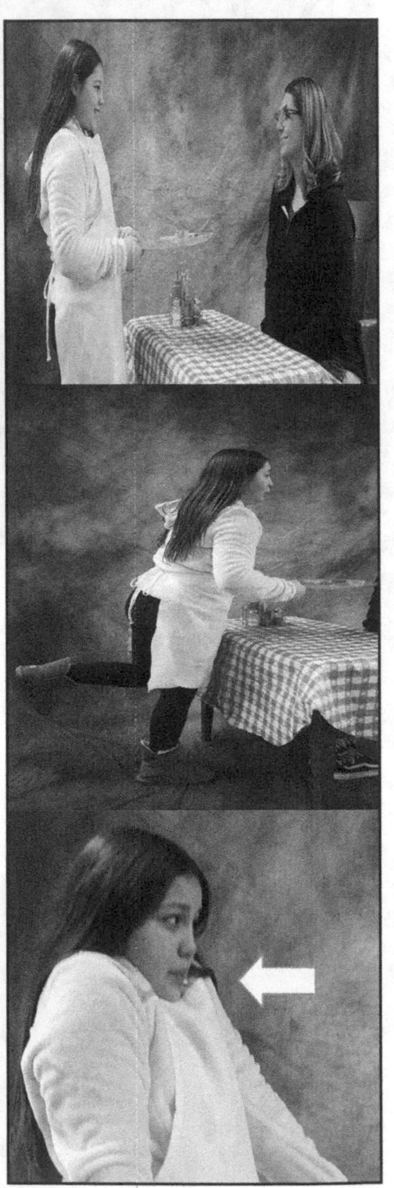

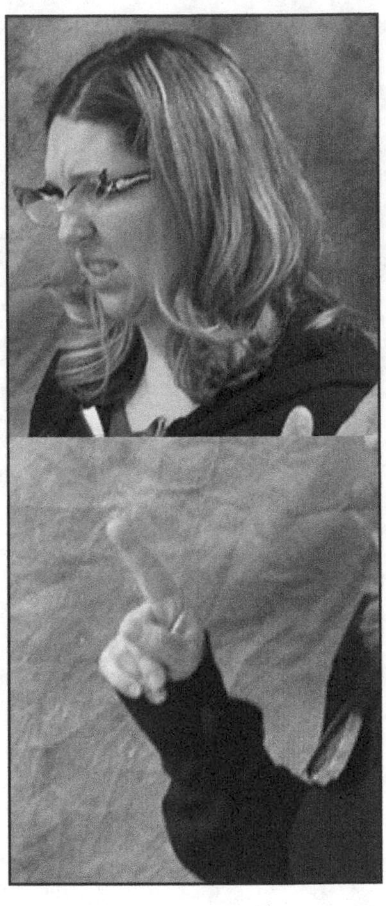

Why Is It Funny?

- Did someone REALLY get food spilled on him or her? No! If he or she did, it would not be funny!
- Do people really act like this when they slip and when they get food spilled on them? No! The funny faces and big movements are what makes it funny to look at!

Next, we will try "Food Fight"

Two people will pretend to throw pretend spaghetti at one another like in a food fight!

What Does Your Face Do When You Are in a Slapstick Food Fight?

- Eyebrows up, oval mouth, surprised
- Eyebrows down, crescent mouth, sneaky smile
- Eyebrows relaxed, crescent mouth, happy

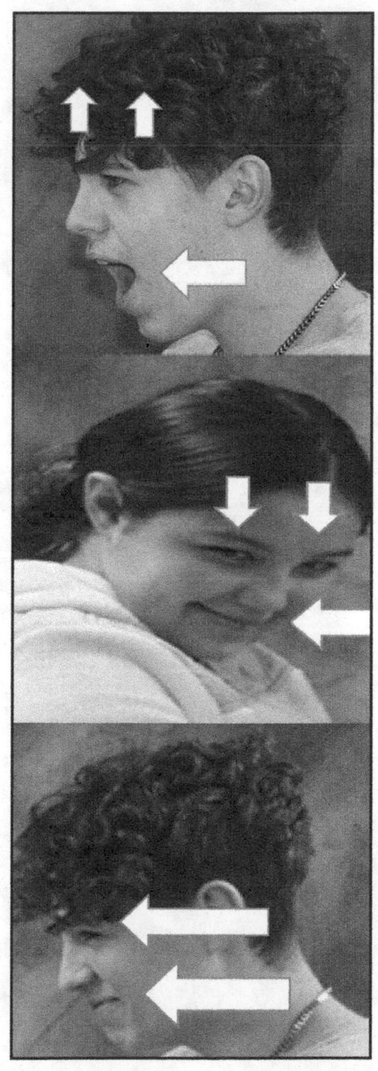

What Does Your Body Do When You Are in a Slapstick Food Fight?

- Arms up in surprise
- Holding food up to throw
- Pointing finger and laughing

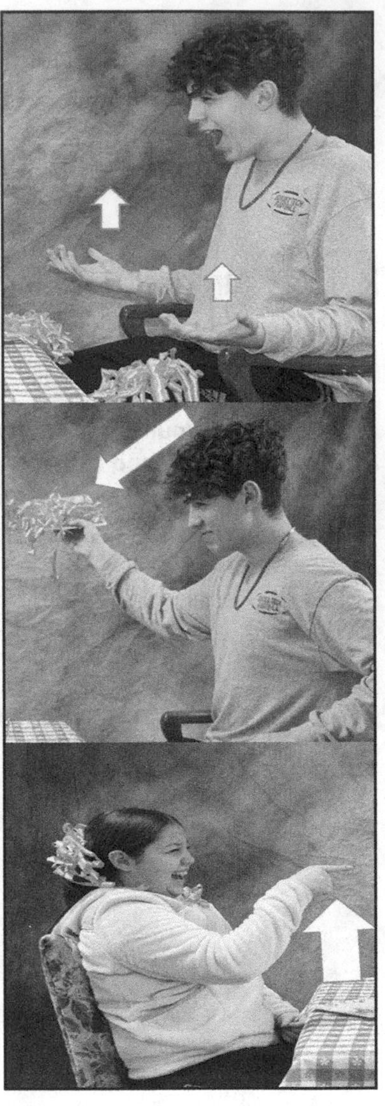

Let's Act Out "Food Fight"

(Both people are seated and have a plate of pretend spaghetti.)

Person 1: Make a sneaky smile and throw some pretend spaghetti at the other person

Person 2: Make a surprised face, then pick up the spaghetti off your plate and throw it at the first person

Person 1: Smile and pick the spaghetti up off yourself/the floor and throw it back at the other person

Person 2: Smile and pick up the spaghetti again and throw it at the first person again

BOTH people look at each other, point, and pretend to laugh at each other

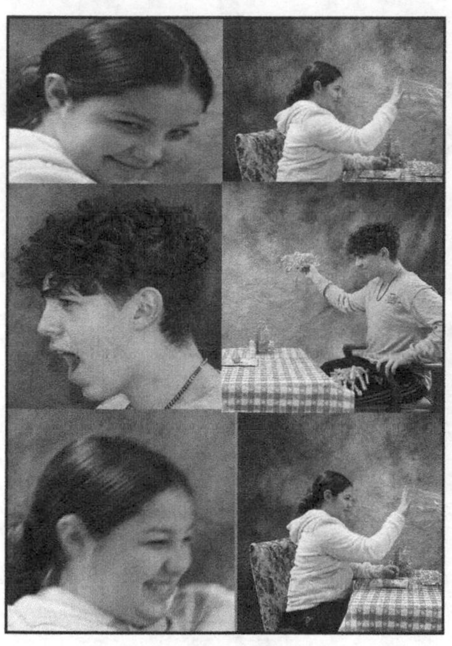

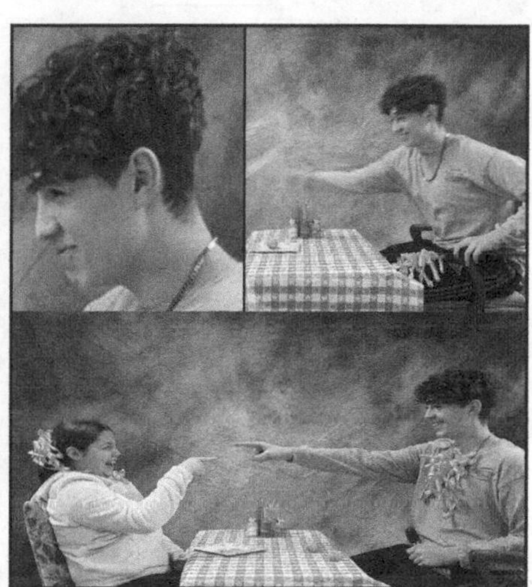

Why Is It Funny?

- Did someone REALLY get in a food fight? No! If they were throwing real food at each other, it might hurt and would make a real mess. It would not be funny!
- Do people really have silly fights like this with real food? No! The silly pretend situation and the funny faces and big movements are what makes it funny!

REVIEW QUESTIONS: MESSY SLAPSTICK

Name:______________________________

1. In "messy slapstick," people may drop or scatter things or do something else to make a ________________.
   A. Cake
   B. Mess
   C. Sweater

2. In real life, you _______ throw food at other people.
   A. Should NOT
   B. Should
   C. Will

3. Is this picture of slapstick or a real mess?
   A. Slapstick
   B. Real mess

4. Is this picture of slapstick or a real mess?
   A. Slapstick
   B. Real mess

5. If someone slipped on food in real life, it ______ be funny.
   A. Would
   B. Should
   C. Would not

Messy Slapstick Review Questions Answer Key

1. B
2. A
3. B
4. A
5. C

CHAPTER 6

Incongruency

Lesson 1: Funny Animals

Objectives

The participant may:

- Increase awareness of incongruity in silly animal pictures
- Understand how incongruity in silly animal pictures can be funny, which can be generalized to finding other types of media humorous (e.g., movies or books with funny animal characters)

Background

At about 4 years of age, children are able to begin telling the difference between what is real and what is imaginary (Malik & Marwaha, 2019). This is important in order for children to progress to McGhee's Stage 3 of humor development, as children find enjoyment in the visual inconsistencies of fantasy books or movies with such themes as anthropomorphism, or animals acting in ways that humans would act (Vogl, 1982). Beginning to identify and resolve incongruities is also essential because it is the foundation for understanding more complex forms of humor later on in development (Samson, 2013). This lesson encourages participants to begin to identify the incongruities in different silly animal pictures and understand why they are funny.

Materials

- Funny Animals Visual Story
- Review Questions and Answer Key
- Animal cutouts page
- Scissors
- Gluesticks
- Blank pieces of paper, two per participant
- Magazines

Preparation

- Use the book or photocopy and staple together the visual story entitled Funny Animals
- Photocopy Review Questions, one for each participant
- Make a copy of animal cutouts, one for each participant

Procedure

- Read the visual story to the participants or have them take turns reading each page. When there are questions, be sure to engage the participants and allow them to answer using their specific mode of communication (speech, communication device, sign language, gestures, etc.). For participants who seem to have a good basic understanding of the concepts in this lesson, ask more challenging questions that make the material more relatable, such as, "Have you ever seen an animal in a cartoon or a book that talks or does something else that animal does not usually do? Give an example."
- For the silly animal cut/paste activity, encourage the participants to complete themselves, but provide assistance for cutting out the props and clothing and making the silly picture, as needed.
- Follow up the activity by having each participant answer the Review Questions, providing assistance as needed. After the participant(s) has completed the questions, the answers given can be compared with the Answer Key.
- Extension activities for this lesson could be:
    - Showing the participants various books or video clips of animals acting like people (e.g., most Disney movies, many children's books)

References

Malik, F., & Marwaha, R. (2019). *Developmental stages of social emotional development in children.* StatPearls Publishing.

Samson, A. (2013). Humor(lessness) elucidated—Sense of humor in individuals with autism spectrum disorders: Review and introduction. *Humor, 26*(3), 393-409.

Vogl, S. (1982). Animals in children's literature. *Wisconsin Academy of Sciences, Arts and Letters, 70*, 68-72.

EXERCISE: FUNNY ANIMALS

Sometimes, in books, movies, or funny pictures called *memes*, animals are shown doing things that they do not normally do.

Today, we are going to talk about photos of animals doing things they do not normally do. This can be funny!

First, let's think—what does a cow normally do?

- Stands
- Eats grass
- Says: "MOOOO!"

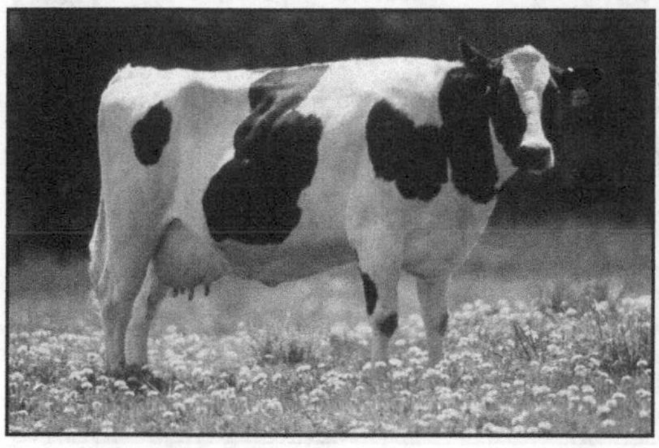

What Else Does a Cow Do?

It is funny to think of a cow doing something a person usually does!

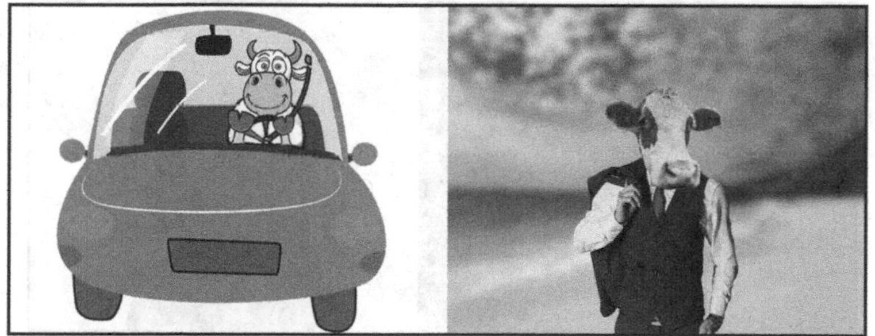

What Is the Cow Doing in These Pictures?

- Do cows usually do this?
- Who normally does this?
- Why is this funny?

What does a dog usually do?

- Walk
- Play with a toy
- Says: "BARK BARK!"

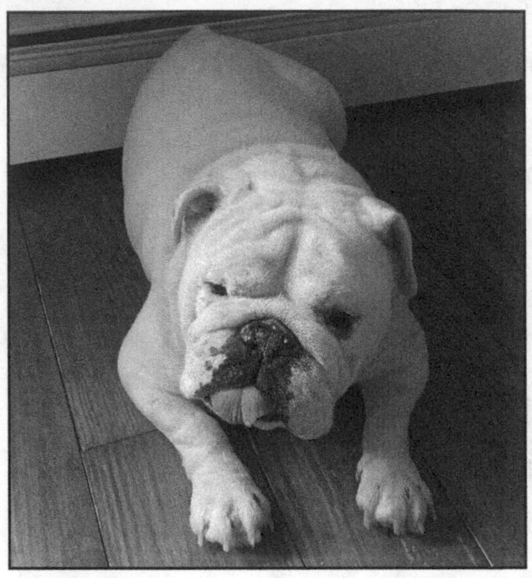

What Else Does a Dog Do?

It is funny to think of a dog doing something a person usually does!

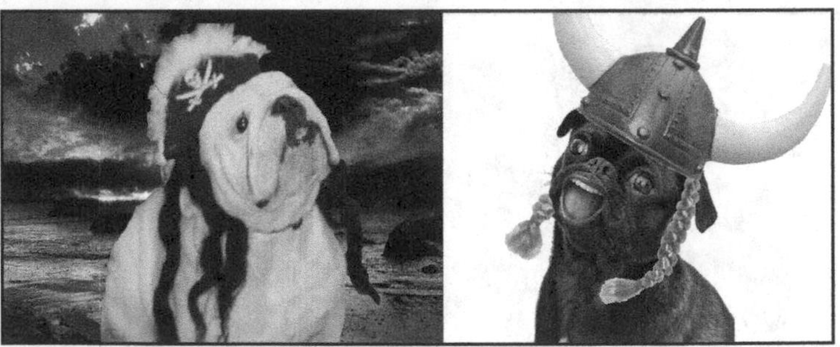

What Is the Dog Doing in These Pictures?

- Do dogs usually do this?
- Who normally does this?
- Why is this funny?

What does a fish usually do?

- Swim
- Make bubbles
- Eat

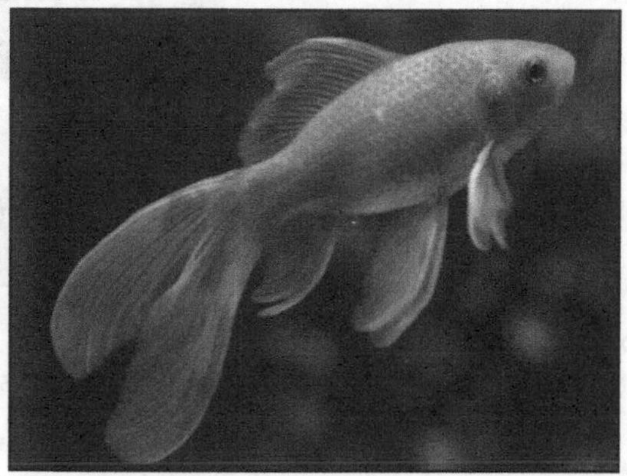

What Else Does a Fish Do?

It is funny to think of a fish doing something a person usually does!

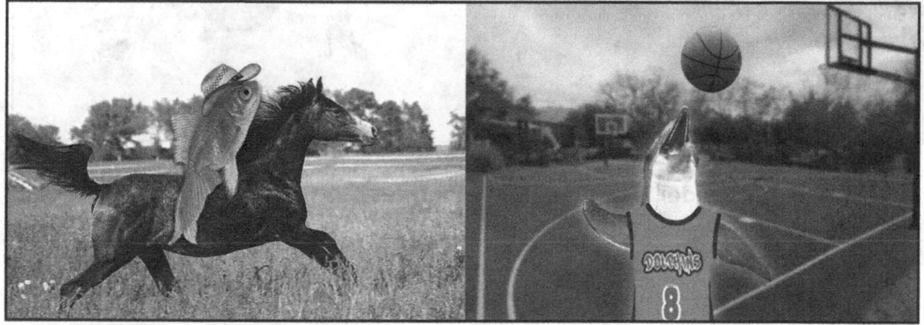

What Is the Fish Doing in These Pictures?

- Do fish usually do this?
- Who normally does this?
- Why is this funny?

What does a spider usually do?

- Spin a web
- Crawl around
- Catch and eat flies

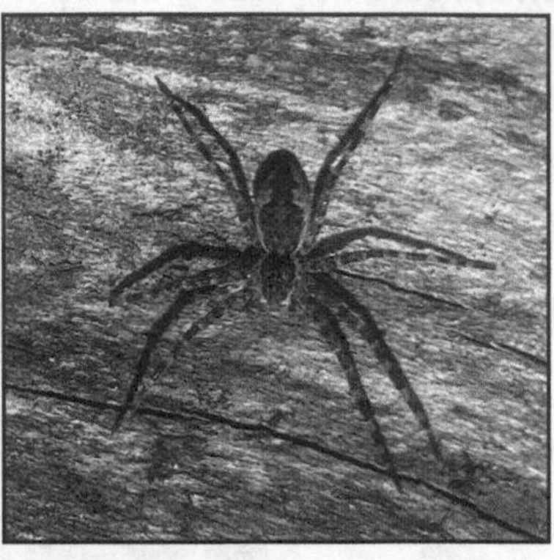

What Else Does a Spider Do?

It is funny to think of a spider doing something a person usually does!

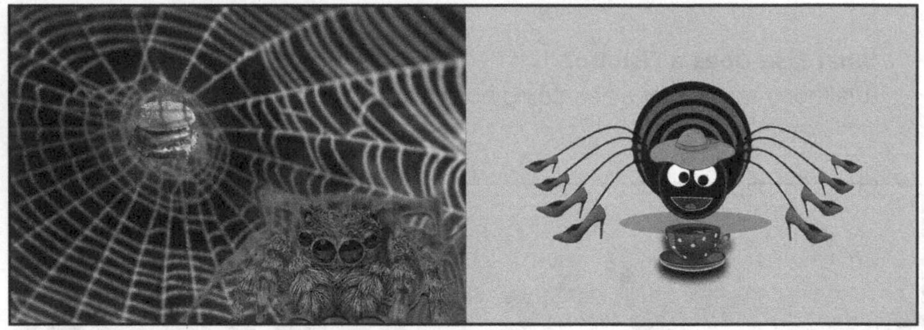

What Is the Spider Doing in These Pictures?

- Do spiders usually do this?
- Who normally does this?
- Why is this funny?

Let's make our own silly pictures!

Find props and clothing in magazines and then cut and paste them on the cow and fish to make them:

- Do something they do not usually do
- Wear something they do not usually wear
- Make a funny face

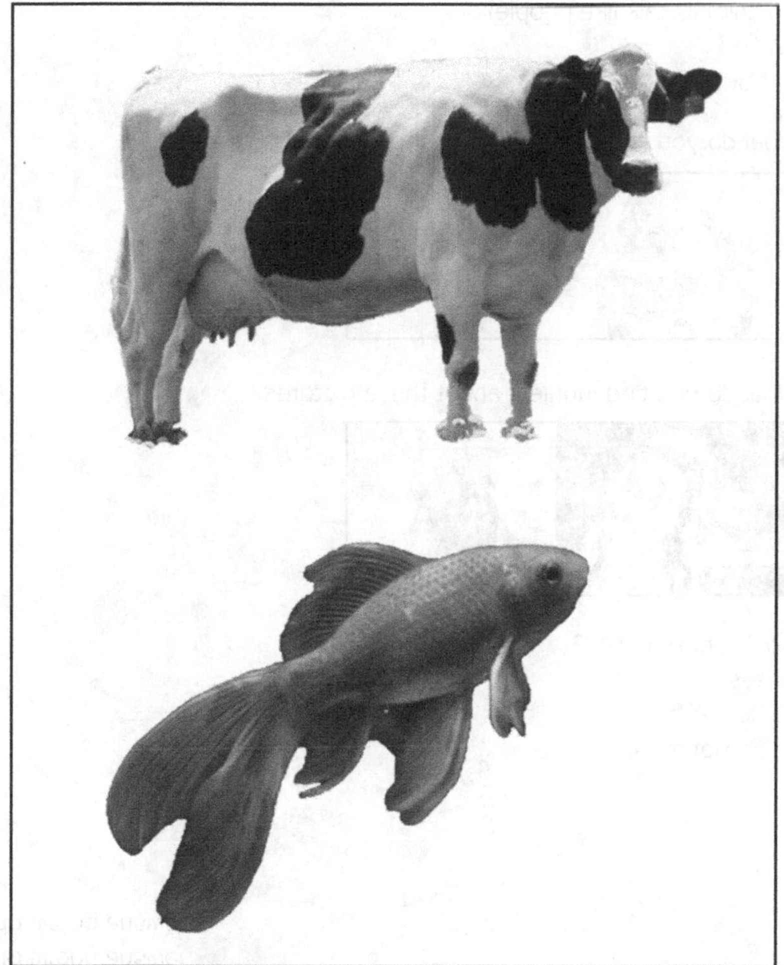

REVIEW QUESTIONS: FUNNY ANIMALS

Name: ______________________________

1. Do animals normally wear clothes?
   A. Yes
   B. No

2. Do animals talk like people?
   A. Yes
   B. No

3. What do you find funniest about these pictures?

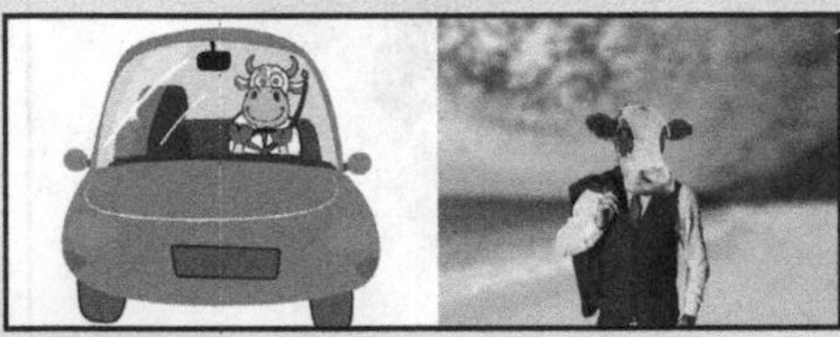

4. What do you find funniest about these pictures?

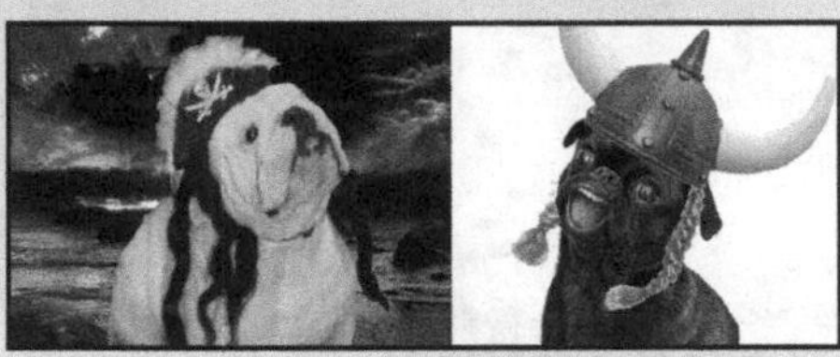

5. Do fish ride horses?
   A. Yes
   B. No
   C. Sometimes

Funny Animals Review Questions Answer Key

1. B
2. B
3. No wrong answer
4. No wrong answer
5. B

Lesson 2: Funny People

Objectives

The participant may:

- Increase awareness of incongruity in silly people pictures
- Understand how incongruity in silly people pictures can be funny, which can be generalized to finding other types of media humorous (e.g., movies or books with funny people characters)

Background

"Visual inconsistencies" are also humorous when people dress and act very differently than a person their age or, better yet, when they act like animals (Southam, 2005). This lesson continues to refine the participant's ability to detect incongruencies in funny photos of babies, older ladies, and other people behaving like animals and improves their understanding of why this is funny.

Materials

- Funny People Visual Story
- Review Questions and Answer Key
- Baby and older lady cutouts page
- Scissors
- Gluesticks
- Blank pieces of paper, three per participant
- Magazines

Preparation

- Use the book or photocopy and staple together the visual story entitled Funny People
- Photocopy Review Questions, one for each participant
- Make a copy of baby/older lady cutout page, one for each participant

Procedure

- Read the visual story to the participants or have them take turns reading each page. When there are questions, be sure to engage the participants and allow them to answer using their specific mode of communication (speech, communication device, sign language, gestures, etc.). For participants who seem to have a good basic understanding of the concepts in this lesson, ask more challenging questions that make the material more relatable, such as, "Have you ever seen a baby in a cartoon or a book that does something only a grown up does? Give an example."
- For the silly people cut/paste activity, encourage the participants to complete themselves, but provide assistance for cutting out the materials and making the silly picture, as needed.
- Follow up the activity by having each participant answer the Review Questions, providing assistance as needed. After the participant(s) has completed the questions, the answers given can be compared with the Answer Key.
- Extension activities for this lesson could be:
    - Showing the participants various books or video clips of babies acting like adults, older people acting much younger, or people acting like animals (e.g., *Boss Baby*, Six Flags commercial featuring dancing older man)

Reference

Southam, M. (2005). Humor development: An important cognitive and social skill in the growing child. *Pediatrics*, 25(1), 105-117.

EXERCISE: FUNNY PEOPLE

Sometimes, in books, movies, or funny pictures called *memes*, people are also shown doing things that they do not normally do.

Today, we are going to talk about photos of different kinds of people doing something they do not normally do. This can be funny!

First, let's think—what does a baby usually do?

- Cry
- Use a rattle
- Drink from a bottle

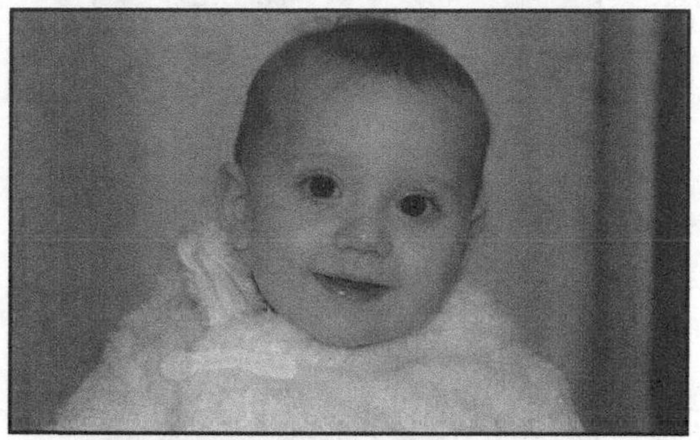

What Else Does a Baby Do?

It is funny to think of a baby doing something an adult would do!

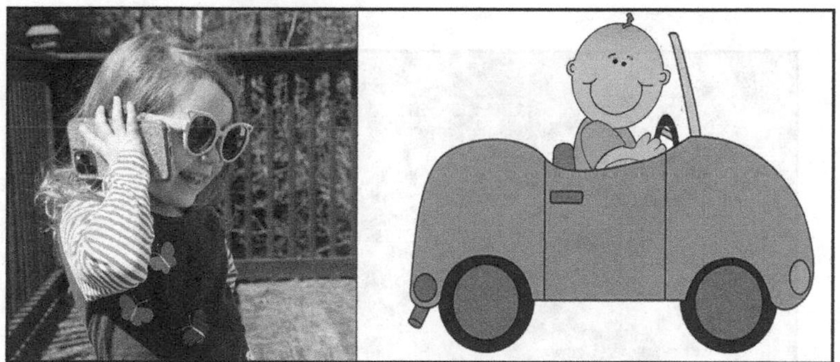

What Is the Baby Doing in These Pictures?

- Do babies usually do this?
- Who normally does this?
- Why is this funny?

What does an older lady usually do?

- Sit in rocker chair
- Walk slowly
- Wear glasses

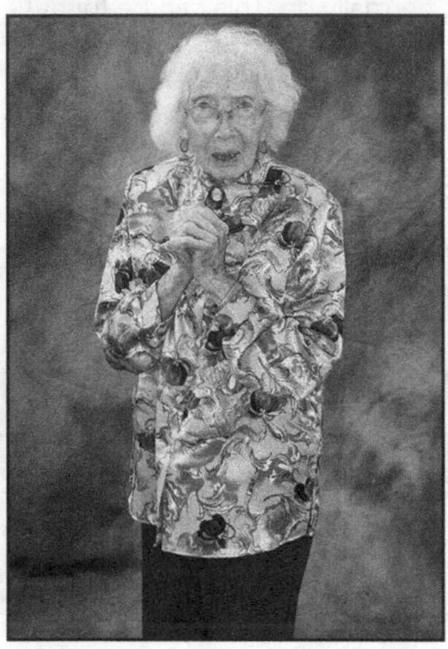

What Else Does an Older Lady Do?

It is funny to think of an older lady doing something a younger person would do!

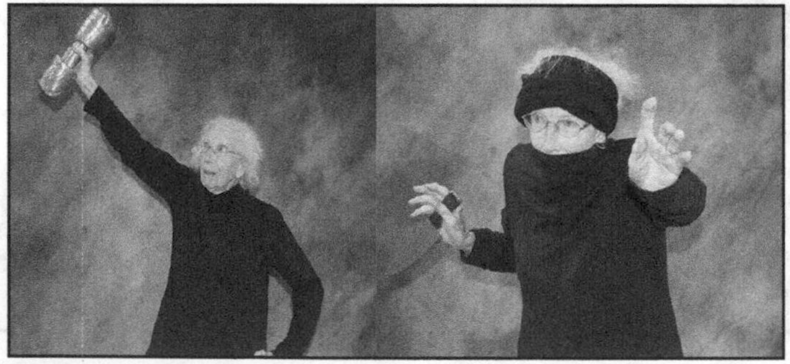

What Is the Older Lady Doing in These Pictures?

- Do older ladies usually do this?
- Who normally does this?
- Why is this funny?

What if we think about people doing things an animal usually does?

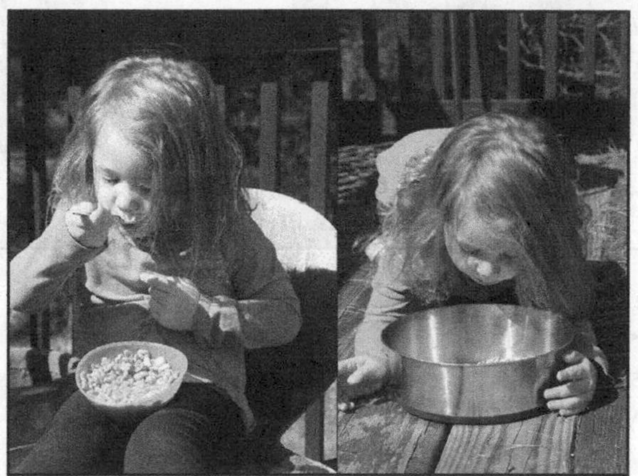

Which One Is Funny?

- Do people eat out of a dish on the floor?
- Who eats out of a dish on the floor?
- Is this funny to think about?

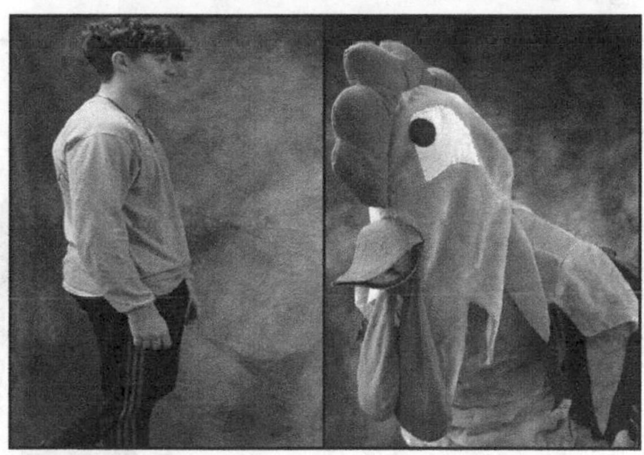

Which One Is Funny?

- Do people have wings and beaks?
- Do people walk with their necks out?
- Is this funny to think about?

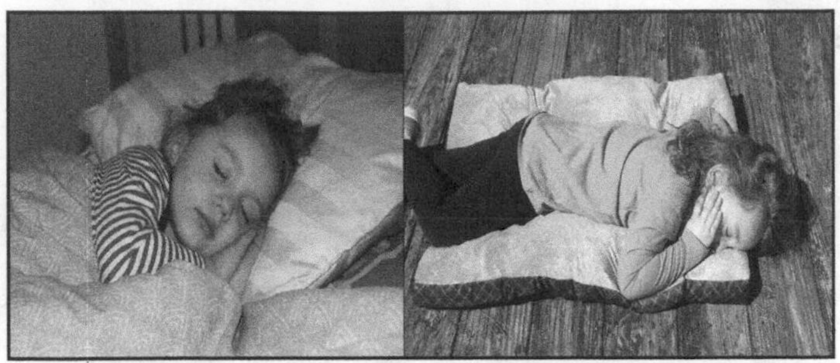

Which One Is Funny?

- Do people sleep on the floor?
- Who sleeps on the floor?
- Is this funny to think about?

Let's make our own funny pictures!

Find props and clothing in magazines and then cut and paste them on the baby and older lady cutouts to make them:

- Do something they do not usually do
- Wear something they do not usually wear
- Do something an animal does

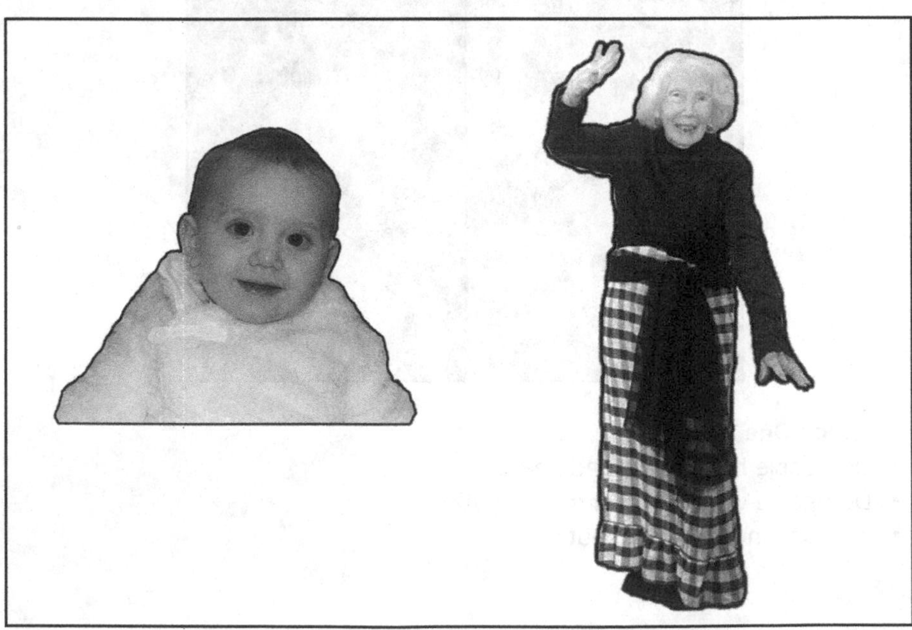

REVIEW QUESTIONS: FUNNY PEOPLE

Name:______________________________

1. Do babies drive cars?
   A. Yes
   B. No

2. Are older ladies usually ninjas?
   A. Yes
   B. No

3. What is funny about this picture?
   A. The person is doing something they do not usually do
   B. The person is doing something an animal does

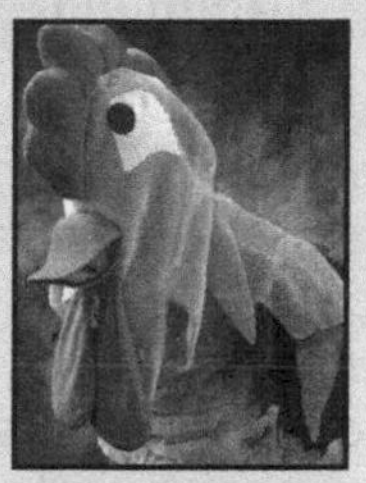

4. What is funny about this picture?
   A. The person is doing something they do not usually do
   B. The person is doing something an animal does

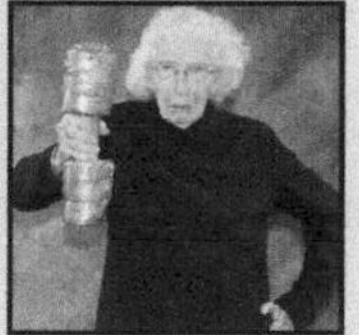

5. How does a person eat cereal?
   A. From a bowl on the ground
   B. With a bowl and fork
   C. With a bowl and spoon

Funny People Review Questions Answer Key

1. B
2. B
3. B
4. A
5. C

Lesson 3: Funny Sizes

Objectives

The participant may:

- Increase awareness of incongruity in the silly objects and costume pieces that clowns use, which are too small or too big
- Understand how incongruity in silly clown prop/costume pictures can be funny

Background

A clown may be considered a master of visual comedy, with his appearance and act being mostly based on visual incongruities. One kind of incongruency clowns use is size incongruency—costume pieces and props that are too small or too big. A clown with a tiny hat, big red nose, and oversized shoes holding a tiny umbrella or oversized hammer can be funny for both children and adults to look at. This lesson encourages participants to identify size incongruities, which can be generalized beyond clowns, and continues to reinforce why visual inconsistencies can be funny.

Materials

- Funny Sizes Visual Story
- Review Questions and Answer Key
- People cutout page (photos of the participants can be used instead)
- Scissors
- Gluesticks
- Blank pieces of paper, two per participant
- Magazines

Preparation

- Use the book or photocopy and staple together the visual story entitled Funny Sizes
- Photocopy Review Questions, one for each participant
- Make a copy of people cutout page, one for each participant (or obtain one photo of each participant)

Procedure

- Read the visual story to the participants or have them take turns reading each page. When there are questions, be sure to engage the participants and allow them to answer using their specific mode of communication (speech, communication device, sign language, gestures, etc.). For participants who seem to have a good basic understanding of the concepts in this lesson, ask more challenging questions that make the material more relatable, such as, "Have you ever seen a clown wear something that did not fit? Have you ever seen a clown use something that was not the right size? Give an example."
- For the funny sizes cut/paste activity, encourage the participants to complete themselves, but provide assistance for cutting out the materials and making the silly picture, as needed.
- Follow up the activity by having each participant answer the Review Questions, providing assistance as needed. After the participant(s) has completed the questions, the answers given can be compared with the Answer Key.
- Extension activities for this lesson could be:
    - Showing the participants various books or video clips of clowns wearing costume pieces and using props that are too big or too small

EXERCISE: FUNNY SIZES

A clown is a performer who dresses up and does different things to be funny. Clowns often have costume pieces or use props that are smaller or bigger than the size of normal objects.

Today, we are going to talk about some of these wrong-sized props and costumes that are funny to look at!

First, let's look at things that are too big. What is too big on this clown?

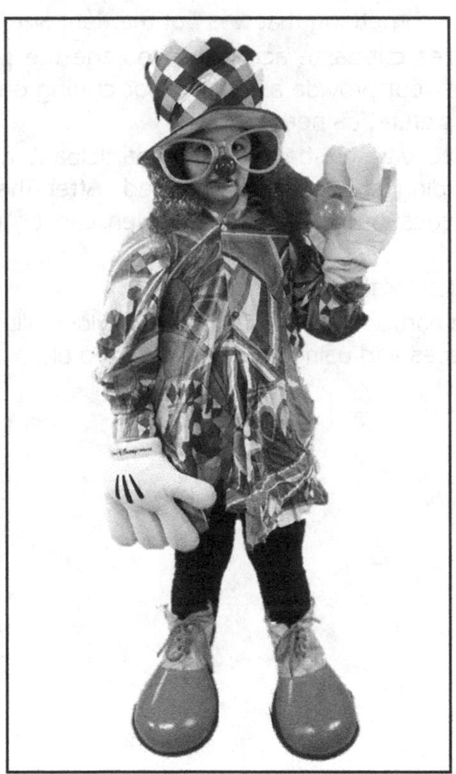

The Shoes

- Do you think the clown's feet are that big? No! She is just wearing them to look funny.
- The clown walks funny because of the big, floppy shoes, which is also funny to watch.

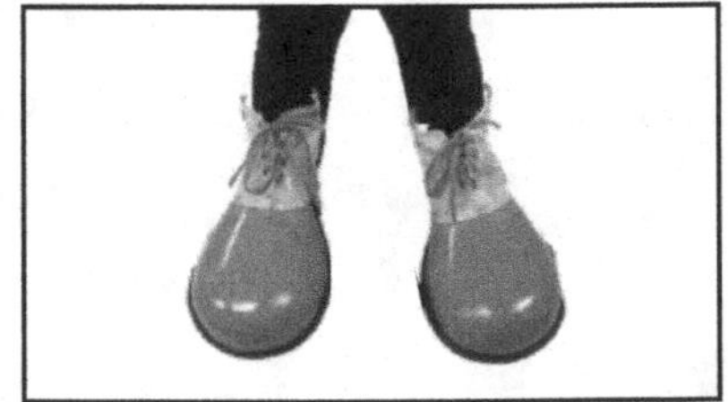

The Hands

- Do you think the clown's hands are that big? No! She is just wearing them to look funny.
- If she tries to do anything with those gloves, it would be tricky, which could be funny to watch.

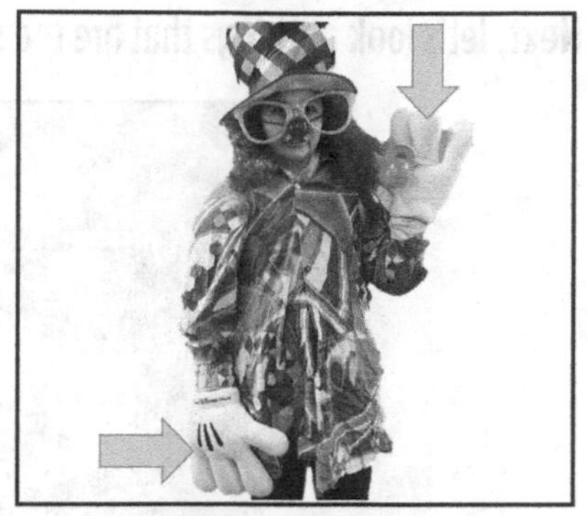

The Glasses

- Do you think the clown's eyes are that big? No! She is just wearing them to look funny.
- If the clown moves her head too much, the glasses will probably fall off, which can also be funny to watch.

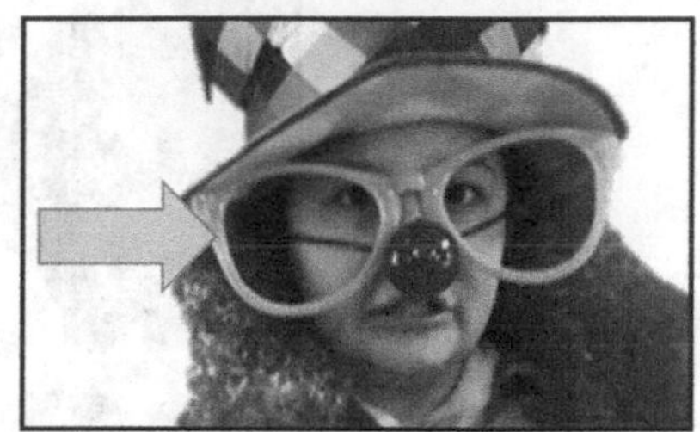

The Hat

- Do you think the clown's head is that big? No! She is just wearing it to look funny.
- If the clown moves her head too much, the hat will probably fall off, which can also be funny to watch.

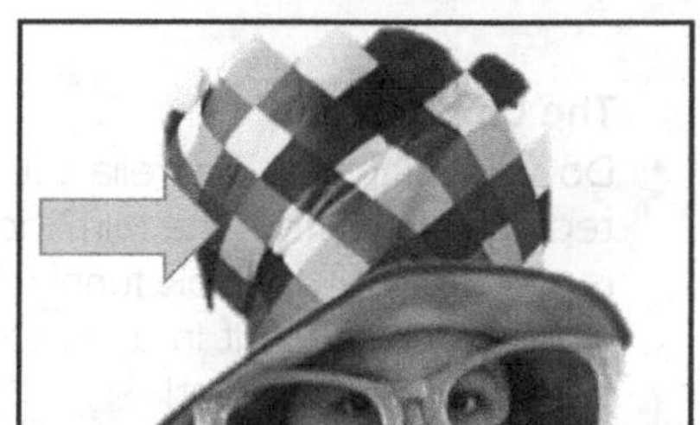

The Nose

- Do you think the clown's nose is that big? Do you think it is really red like that? No! She is just wearing a fake nose to look funny.
- Sometimes, red clown noses also blink or squeak when you squeeze them, which can also be funny to watch and hear.

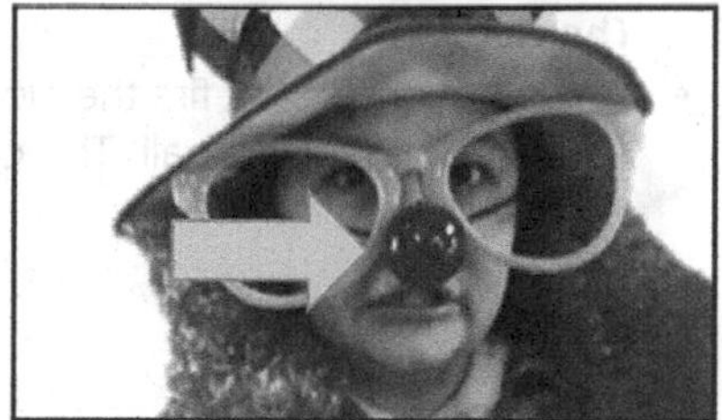

Next, let's look at things that are too small. What is too small for this clown?

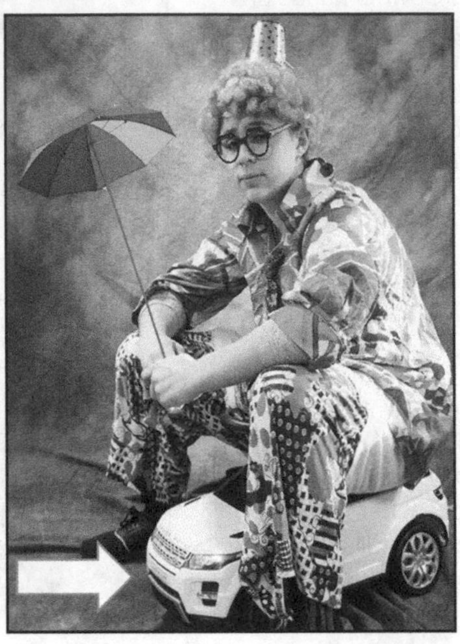

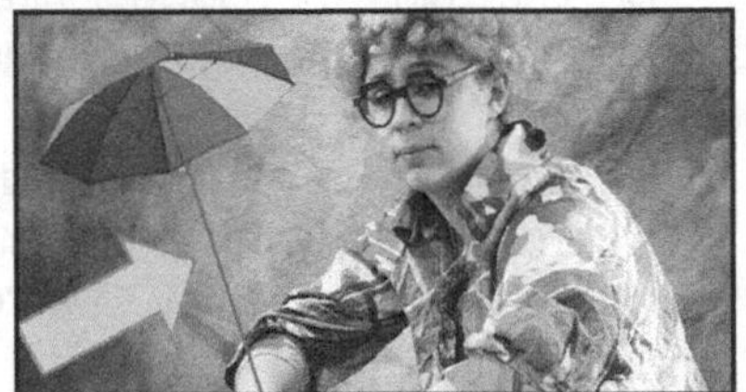

The Umbrella

- Do you think the umbrella will protect the clown from the rain? No! He is just using it to look funny. If he were to really use it in a rainstorm, he would get very wet!

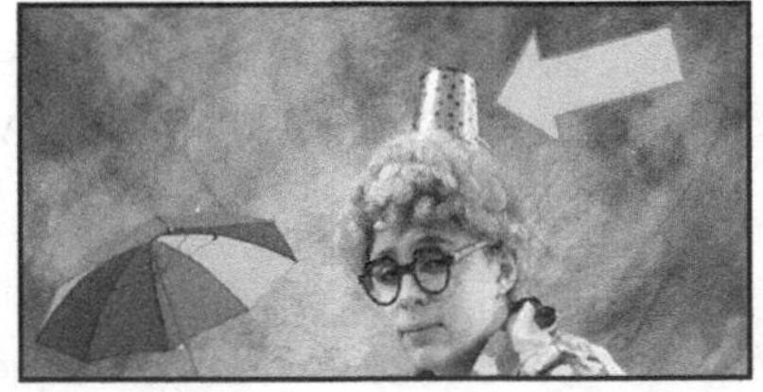

The Hat

- Do you think the hat fits the clown's head? No! It is too small. The clown is wearing it to look funny.

The Car

- Do you think the clown fits well in that car? No! It is too small. When the clown rides it, it looks very funny!

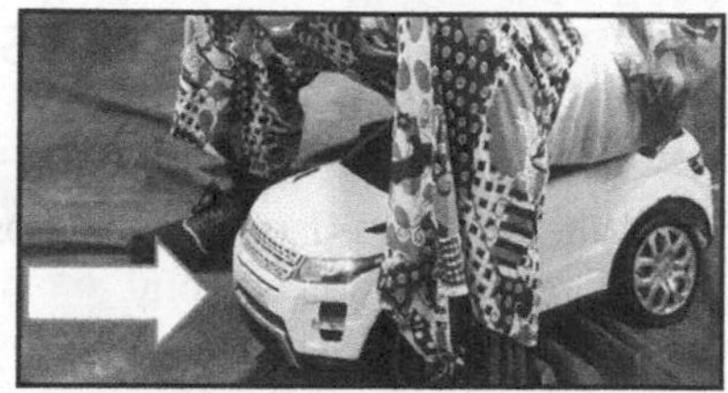

Let's make our own silly pictures!

Find props and clothing in magazines and then cut and paste them on the people cutouts/photos to make them:

- Use something that is the wrong size
- Wear something that is the wrong size

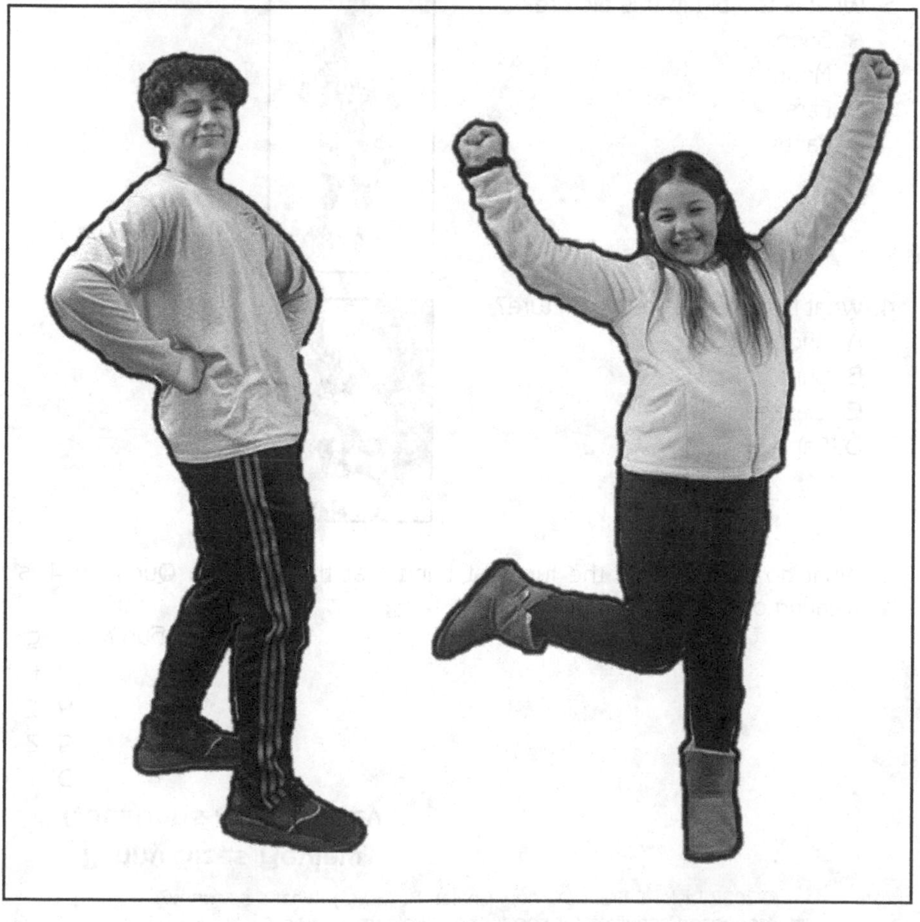

REVIEW QUESTIONS: FUNNY SIZES

Name: ______________________________

1. When clowns use props or costume pieces that are too ________ or too ________, it can be funny.
   A. Colorful, dark
   B. Ugly, pretty
   C. Big, small
   D. Cold, hot

2. Who usually wears clothes or uses props that are too small or too big?
   A. Doctor
   B. Clown
   C. Mailman

3. What is too big in this picture?
   A. Shoes
   B. Mouth
   C. Ears
   D. Pants

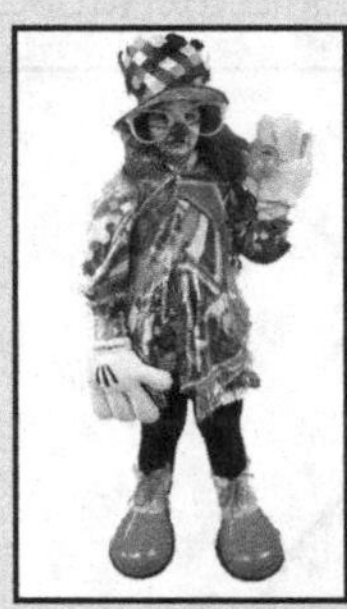

4. What is too small in this picture?
   A. Shoes
   B. Shirt
   C. Glasses
   D. Car

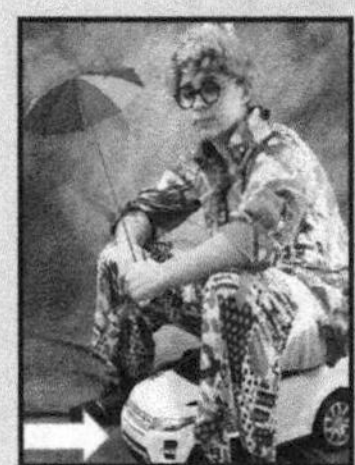

5. What do you think is the funniest thing that the clown in Question 4 is wearing or doing?

Funny Sizes Review Questions Answer Key

1. C
2. B
3. A
4. D
5. No wrong answer

CHAPTER 7

Pranks

Lesson 1: Food Pranks

Objectives

The participant may:

- Improve his or her understanding of what a prank is
- Understand why food pranks are funny
- Understand how a person can use food pranks to be funny and interact with others

Background

By the age of 4 years, most typical-developing children begin to enjoy playfully tricking others and being tricked themselves, like hiding an object behind their back and saying they do not know where it is (Malik & Marwaha, 2019). In Stage 4 of McGhee's humor development, more "malicious" types of humor begin to be enjoyed, such as teasing and pranks (Buijzen & Valkenburg, 2004). Studies have shown that teasing and pranks have been observed to be enjoyed by individuals with intellectual disabilities as much as their neurotypical peers (Chadwick & Platt, 2018). In addition, the food pranks use "sudden visual surprises," which are enjoyable by individuals who have an emerging sense of humor (Buijzen & Valkenburg, 2004).

Materials

- Food Pranks Visual Story
- Review Questions and Answer Key
- Chips can popper
- Ice cream popper

Chaiet, R. *What's So Funny?: Humor-Based Activities for Social Skill Development* (pp. 101-127).

Preparation

- Use the book or photocopy and staple together the visual story entitled Food Pranks
- Photocopy Review Questions, one for each participant
- Purchase the chips can popper and the ice cream popper

Procedure

- Read the visual story to the participants or have them take turns reading each page. When there are questions, be sure to engage the participants and allow them to answer using their specific mode of communication (speech, communication device, sign language, gestures, etc.). For participants who seem to have a good basic understanding of the concepts in this lesson, ask more challenging questions that make the material more relatable, such as, "Have you ever pranked someone? Has someone pranked you? What were the pranks? How did those pranks make you feel?"
- When introducing the pranks, first show them by modeling the prank with another adult, if possible. The adult being pranked should have an exaggerated reaction (i.e., wide eyes and surprised look, arms up, and say "AHHHHHH!"). Then, the participant can try it with an adult, who should, again, have an exaggerated reaction. If the activity is being done with a group, the participant should then try the prank with a peer.
- Follow up the activity by having each participant answer the Review Questions, providing assistance as needed. After the participant(s) has completed the questions, the answers given can be compared with the Answer Key.
- Extension activities for this lesson could be:
  - Showing the participants various video clips of pranks related to food (e.g., YouTube videos of people pranking each other with toothpaste Oreos, pies in the face, exploding soda)

References

Buijzen, M., & Valkenburg, P. (2004). Developing a typology of humor in audiovisual media. *Media Psychology, 6*, 147-167.

Chadwick, D., & Platt, T. (2018). Investigating humor in social interaction in people with intellectual disabilities: A systematic review of the literature. *Frontiers in Psychology, 9*, 1745.

Malik, F., & Marwaha, R. (2019). *Developmental stages of social emotional development in children.* StatPearls Publishing.

EXERCISE: FOOD PRANKS

A prank is a trick that you play on someone to be funny! You usually trick them to think one thing is something else…but then you surprise them!

Today, we are going to play pranks with pretend food. We will offer someone something that looks like food, but when they try to eat it—surprise! It's not!

These food pranks are funny because people may think they are going to get a tasty treat and then something unexpected happens!

Chips Prank

You are going to offer a person some of your chips. When they go to open them, a pretend snake will pop out at them! Surprise!

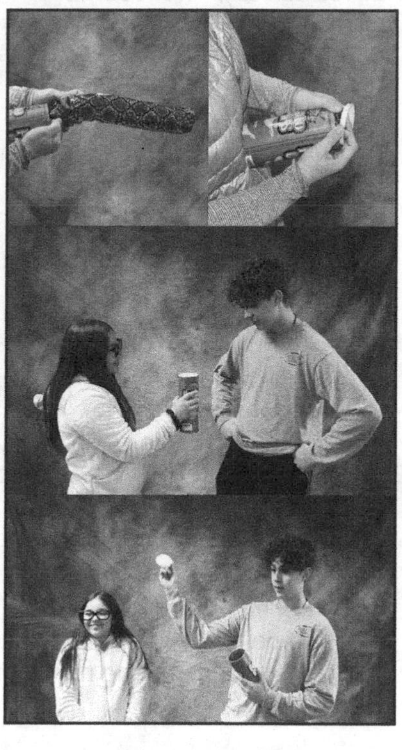

Prank Steps

1. Make sure snake is in can and top is on container.
2. Hand the person the can. You can say "Want some?" and have them open the can.
3. The snake will pop out! Surprise!

How Did It Go?

- Did the person smile/laugh?
  Yes No
- Did you smile or laugh?
  Yes No
- Did you think it was funny?
  Yes No

Why Is It Funny?

- Does a snake usually pop out of a can of chips? No! The person being pranked was expecting to just eat some chips, and a fake snake popped out at them instead.
- Because it was not what they expected, this can be funny for the person being pranked.
- It can be funny for the prankster to watch the reaction of the person being pranked, as they may jump back and make a funny face!

Ice Cream Popper Prank

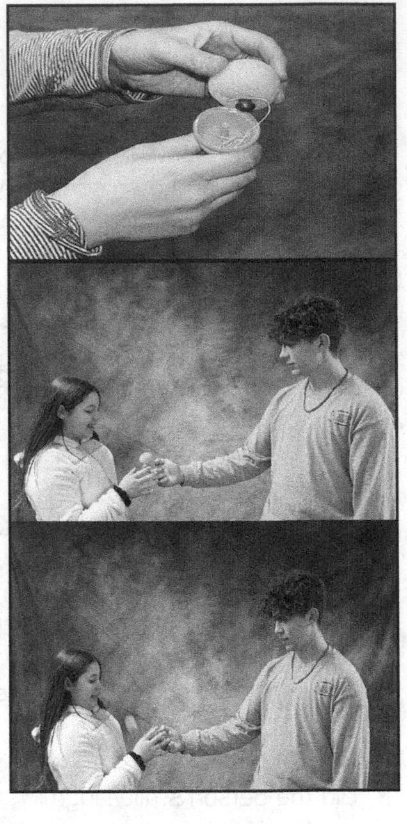

You are going to offer a person some of your ice cream. You will then push a button for the top of the ice cream to pop off. Surprise!

Prank Steps

1. Make sure ice cream top is on and string is tucked inside cone.
2. You can say, "Want some?"
3. As they go to take it, push the button to pop the ice cream in the air!

How Did It Go?

- Did the person smile/laugh?
  Yes No
- Did you smile or laugh?
  Yes No
- Did you think it was funny?
  Yes No

Why Is It Funny?

- Does the top of ice cream really pop off like that? No! The person being pranked was expecting to just eat some ice cream, and it popped out at him or her instead.
- Because it was not what he or she expected, this can be funny for the person being pranked.
- It can be funny for the prankster to watch the reaction of the person being pranked, as he or she may jump back and make a funny face!

REVIEW QUESTIONS: FOOD PRANKS

Name:______________________________

1. Does a snake usually pop out of a chip container in real life?
   A. Yes
   B. No
   C. Sometimes

2. Does ice cream usually pop out at you in real life?
   A. Yes
   B. No
   C. Sometimes

3. A prank is a _____ you play on someone to be funny.
   A. Trick
   B. Secret
   C. Chore

4. A prank is funny because something ________ happens.
   A. Cool
   B. Mean
   C. Unexpected

5. It can also be funny to see the person's ________ to the prank.
   A. Reaction
   B. Fingers
   C. Cry

Food Pranks Review Questions Answer Key

1. B
2. B
3. A
4. C
5. A

Lesson 2: Water Pranks

Objectives

The participant may:

- Understand why water pranks are funny
- Understand how a person can use water pranks to be funny and interact with others

Background

From water guns to playing in a hose, many children and adolescents enjoy a little water play from time to time. In addition to being visual in nature, these pranks add the tactile component of water for a fun, multisensory activity, including the classic clown squirting flower prank. Multisensory experiences have been shown to increase engagement and enjoyment of activities for individuals with disabilities, meaning these pranks should be doubly enjoyed by all participants (Metcalf et al., 2009).

Materials

- Water Pranks Visual Story
- Review Questions and Answer Key
- Squirting ring
- Squirting flower

Preparation

- Use the book or photocopy and staple together the visual story entitled Water Pranks
- Photocopy Review Questions, one for each participant
- Purchase the squirting ring and squirting flower
- Have water available for both pranks

Procedure

- Read the visual story to the participants or have them take turns reading each page. When there are questions, be sure to engage the participants and allow them to answer using their specific mode of communication (speech, communication device, sign language, gestures, etc.). For participants who seem to have a good basic understanding of the concepts in this lesson, ask more challenging questions that make the material more relatable, such as, "Have you ever seen a clown with a squirting flower? Have you ever been squirted with water unexpectedly? How did it make you feel?"
- When introducing the pranks, first show them by modeling the prank with another adult, if possible. The adult being pranked should have an exaggerated reaction (i.e., wide eyes and surprised look, arms up, and say "AHHHHHH!"). Then, the participant can try it with an adult, who should, again, have an exaggerated reaction. If the activity is being done with a group, the participant should then try the prank with a peer.
- Follow up the activity by having each participant answer the Review Questions, providing assistance as needed. After the participant(s) has completed the questions, the answers given can be compared with the Answer Key.
- Extension activities for this lesson could be:
  - Showing the participants various video clips of pranks related to water (e.g., YouTube videos of people pranking each other with water guns, buckets of water, and other squirting toy pranks)

Reference

Metcalf, D., Evans, C., Flynn, H. K., & Williams, J. B. (2009). Direct instruction + UDL = Access for diverse learners: How to plan and implement an effective multisensory spelling lesson. *Teaching Exceptional Children Plus*, 5(6), Article 2.

EXERCISE: WATER PRANKS

Today, we are going to play pranks with water. You will show someone something that looks like a common object, but then it will shoot water at them. Surprise!

Squirting Ring Prank

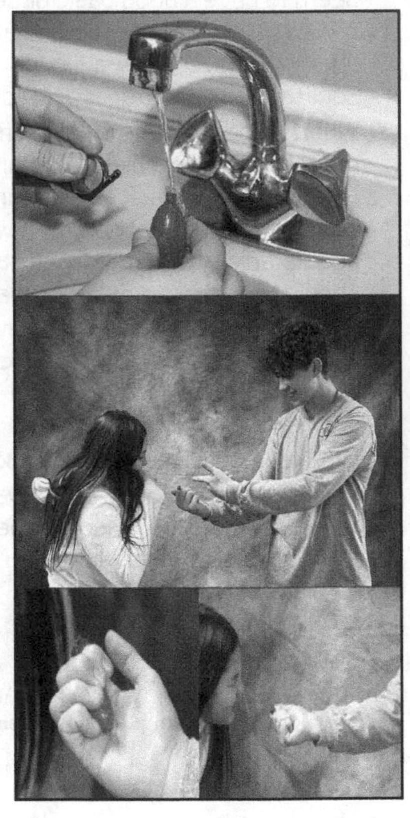

You are going to show a person your ring. When they go to look at it, you squirt water at them! Surprise!

Prank Steps

1. Make sure the bulb attached to the ring is full of water.
2. Show the person your ring. You can say "Look at my ring!"
3. Squeeze the bulb to squirt them with water! Surprise!

How Did It Go?

- Did the person smile/laugh?
  Yes No
- Did you smile or laugh?
  Yes No
- Did you think it was funny?
  Yes No

Why Is It Funny?

- Does water usually squirt out of a ring? No! The person being pranked was expecting to just look at the ring, but then water squirted at him or her instead.
- Because it was not what he or she expected, this can be funny for the person being pranked.
- It can be funny for the prankster to watch the reaction of the person being pranked, as he or she may jump back and make a funny face!

Squirting Flower Prank

You are going to show someone a flower and ask him or her to smell it. When the person does, you will squeeze a bulb that makes the flower shoot water. Surprise!

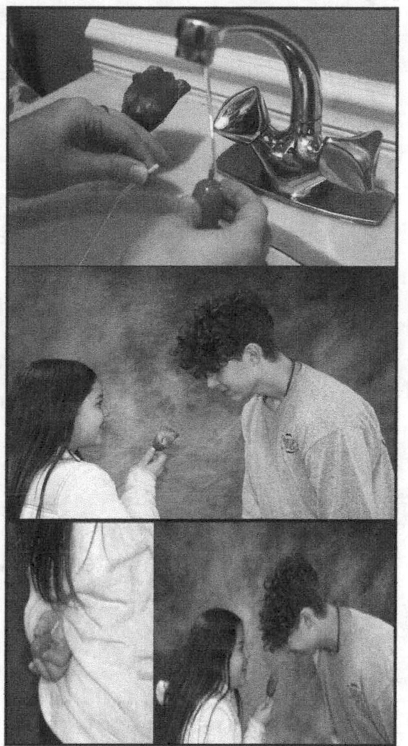

Prank Steps

1. Make sure bulb base connected to flower stem is full of water.
2. You can say to someone "Smell my flower!"
3. Once they get close to the flower, squeeze the bulb to squirt them with water! Surprise!

How Did It Go?

- Did the person smile/laugh?
  Yes No
- Did you smile or laugh?
  Yes No
- Did you think it was funny?
  Yes No

Why Is It Funny?

- Does water usually squirt out of a flower? No! The person being pranked was expecting to just smell the flower, but then water squirted at him or her instead.
- Because it was not what he or she expected, this can be funny for the person being pranked.
- It can be funny for the prankster to watch the reaction of the person being pranked, as he or she may jump back and make a funny face!

REVIEW QUESTIONS: WATER PRANKS

Name: ______________________________

1. Does a ring usually squirt water at you in real life?
   A. Yes
   B. No
   C. Sometimes

2. Does a flower usually squirt water at you in real life?
   A. Yes
   B. No
   C. Sometimes

3. When you play a prank on someone, you want him or her to:
   A. Smile/laugh
   B. Cry
   C. Yell

4. Before you start a water prank, you should make sure the prank is full of:
   A. Dirt
   B. Candy
   C. Water

5. Should you squirt someone in the eyes with a water prank?
   A. No
   B. Yes
   C. Sometimes

Water Pranks Review Questions Answer Key

1. B
2. B
3. A
4. C
5. A

Lesson 3: Bug Pranks

Objectives

The participant may:

- Understand why bug pranks are funny
- Understand how a person can use bug pranks to be funny and interact with others

Background

Many children enjoy creepy things, like bugs or scary stories, as long as they know they are in a safe environment (Ringo, 2013). One reason for this may be because many people experience a release of dopamine when they watch or experience something scary. In addition, individuals who enjoy activities that make them a little scared have an opportunity to practice overcoming negative emotions. These bug pranks provide just the right amount of a fear factor to pique the interest of participants, while affording them the opportunity to use them to interact with others.

Materials

- Bug Pranks Visual Story
- Review Questions and Answer Key
- Small fake fly
- Fake rolling cockroach
- Fake spider
- Ice cube tray (optional)
- Thin white thread
- Cup of water

Preparation

- Use the book or photocopy and staple together the visual story entitled Bug Pranks
- Photocopy Review Questions, one for each participant
- Purchase fake fly, fake rolling cockroach, and fake spider
- *Optional*: Make a "fly ice cube" by putting it in a filled up ice cube tray overnight
- Tie thread around fake spider's body
- Fill a cup with water

Procedure

- Read the visual story to the participants or have them take turns reading each page. When there are questions, be sure to engage the participants and allow them to answer using their specific mode of communication (speech, communication device, sign language, gestures, etc.). For participants who seem to have a good basic understanding of the concepts in this lesson, ask more challenging questions that make the material more relatable, such as, "Are you afraid of bugs? Has a bug ever jumped out and scared you? Have you ever had a bug in your food? How did that make you feel?"
- When introducing the pranks, first show them by modeling the prank with another adult, if possible. The adult being pranked should have an exaggerated reaction (i.e., wide eyes and surprised look, arms up, and say "AHHHHHH!"). Then, the participant can try it with an adult, who should, again, have an exaggerated reaction. If the activity is being done with a group, the participant should then try the prank with a peer.
- Follow up the activity by having each participant answer the Review Questions, providing assistance as needed. After the participant(s) has completed the questions, the answers given can be compared with the Answer Key.
- Extension activities for this lesson could be:
  - Showing the participants various video clips of pranks related to bugs (e.g., YouTube videos of people pranking each other with fake or real bugs)

Reference

Ringo, A. (2013, October 31). Why do some brains enjoy fear?: The science behind the appeal of haunted houses, freak shows and physical thrills. *The Atlantic*. https://www.theatlantic.com/health/archive/2013/10/why-do-some-brains-enjoy-fear/280938/

EXERCISE: BUG PRANKS

Today, we are going to do pranks that have to do with bugs. People will think that a bug is near them, but then they will realize it is fake. Surprise!

Fly in a Drink Prank

You are going to offer a person a glass of water. When he or she goes to drink it, there will be a fake fly in the drink! Surprise!

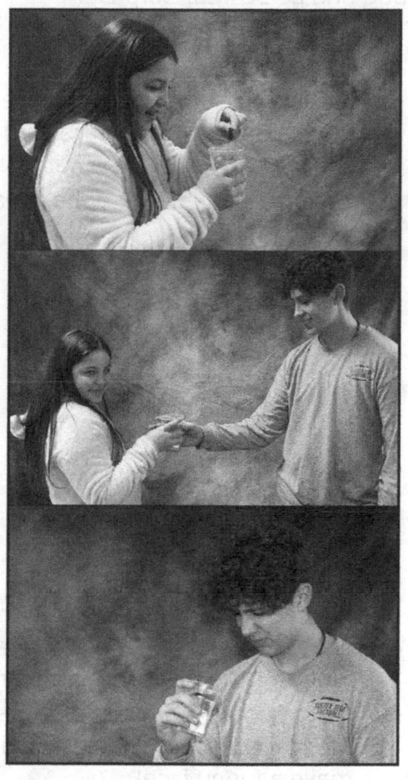

Prank Steps

1. Get a cup of water and put a fake fly in it. You can also use a fly that you have frozen in an ice cube the day before.
2. Hand the person the cup.
3. When he or she goes to take a drink, he or she will see the fly! Yuck! Surprise!

How Did It Go?

- Did the person smile/laugh?
  Yes No
- Did you smile or laugh?
  Yes No
- Did you think it was funny?
  Yes No

Why Is It Funny?

- Are flies usually in your drink? No! The person being pranked was expecting to just take a drink of clean water, but he or she had a gross fly in there instead.
- Because it was not what he or she expected, and because it is a little bit scary, this can be funny for the person being pranked.
- Many people are afraid of bugs. It can be funny for the prankster to watch the reaction of the person being pranked, as he or she may jump back and make a funny face!

Rolling Cockroach Prank

You are going to roll a fake cockroach toward a person. When he or she sees it, the person will think it is a real bug and be scared. Surprise!

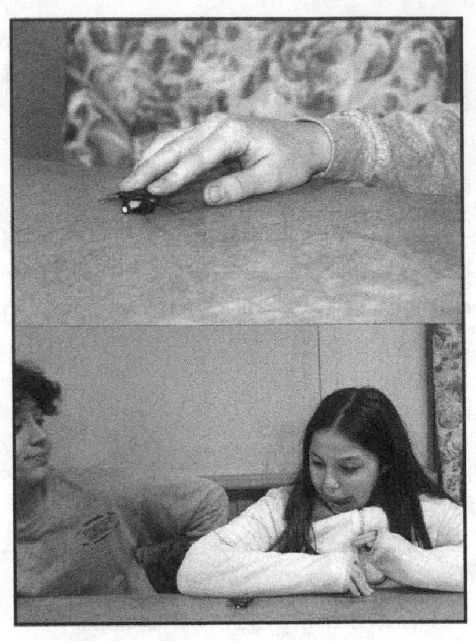

Prank Steps

1. Sit next to someone at a table and roll the fake cockroach toward him or her when he or she is not looking.
2. Watch how he or she reacts. Surprise!

How Did It Go?

- Did the person smile/laugh?
  Yes No
- Did you smile or laugh?
  Yes No
- Did you think it was funny?
  Yes No

Why Is It Funny?

- Are cockroaches usually crawling on the table toward us? No! Because it was not what he or she expected, and because it is a little bit scary, this can be funny for the person being pranked.
- Many people are afraid of bugs. It can be funny for the prankster to watch the reaction of the person being pranked, as he or she may jump back and make a funny face!

Spider on a String Prank

You are going to put a fake spider on a string and make it land on someone's shoulder. When the person sees it, he or she will think it is a real spider and be scared. Surprise!

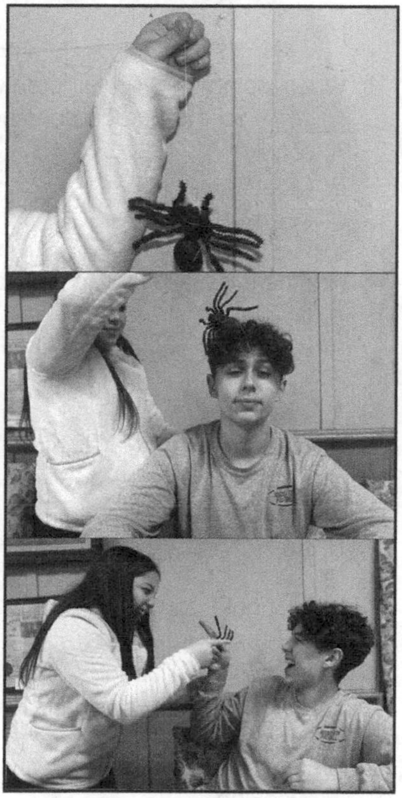

Prank Steps

1. Make sure a string is tightly tied to your fake spider.
2. Quietly come up behind someone so he or she cannot see you. Slowly lower the spider onto the person's shoulder.
3. Watch how the person reacts. Surprise!

How Did It Go?

- Did the person smile/laugh?
  Yes No
- Did you smile or laugh?
  Yes No
- Did you think it was funny?
  Yes No

Why Is It Funny?

- Do big spiders usually land on your shoulder? No! Because it was not what he or she expected, and because it is a little bit scary, this can be funny for the person being pranked.
- Many people are afraid of bugs. It can be funny for the prankster to watch the reaction of the person being pranked, as he or she may jump back and make a funny face!

REVIEW QUESTIONS: BUG PRANKS

Name:______________________________

1. When doing the spider prank, you should come up behind the person _______ so the person does not see or hear you before the prank.
   A. Loudly
   B. Quietly
   C. Cranky

2. Are there usually flies in your drink?
   A. No
   B. Yes
   C. Always

3. If someone is extremely afraid of bugs, should you play bug pranks on him or her?
   A. Yes
   B. No

4. Why should you not play a prank on someone who is extremely afraid of bugs?
   A. He or she will laugh
   B. He or she may be scared

5. When you do the rolling cockroach prank, you should wait until the person ___ looking.
   A. Is
   B. Is not

Bug Pranks Review Questions Answer Key

1. B
2. A
3. B
4. B
5. B

Lesson 4: Gross Pranks

Objectives

The participant may:

- Understand why gross pranks can be funny
- Understand how a person can use gross pranks to be funny and interact with others

Background

Whether we like it or not, potty jokes play a part in humor development. Pranks involving bodily functions, like farting and pooping, can be enjoyable and motivating for individuals who have an emerging sense of humor, as they involve an unusual sound, and continue to feature an "incongruous and surprising event" (Buijzen & Valkenburg, 2004, p. 150). These pranks can also be amusing to an older, adolescent crowd who may prefer humor "based on taboos or disgust" (Buijzen & Valkenburg, 2004, p. 150).

Materials

- Gross Pranks Visual Story
- Review Questions and Answer Key
- Whoopee cushion
- Fake dog poop

Preparation

- Use the book or photocopy and staple together the visual story entitled Gross Pranks
- Photocopy Review Questions, one for each participant
- Purchase the whoopee cushion and fake dog poop

Procedure

- Read the visual story to the participants or have them take turns reading each page. When there are questions, be sure to engage the participants and allow them to answer using their specific mode of communication (speech, communication device, sign language, gestures, etc.). For participants who seem to have a good basic understanding of the concepts in this lesson, ask more challenging questions that make the material more relatable, such as "Do you think it is funny when you or someone else passes gas? Is it more funny or embarrassing? Has your dog or cat ever pooped in the house? How did it make you feel?"
- When introducing the pranks, first show them by modeling the prank with another adult, if possible. The adult being pranked should have an exaggerated reaction (i.e., wide eyes and surprised look, arms up, and say "AHHHHHH!"). Then, the participant can try it with an adult, who should, again, have an exaggerated reaction. If the activity is being done with a group, the participant should then try the prank with a peer.
- Follow up the activity by having each participant answer the Review Questions, providing assistance as needed. After the participant(s) has completed the questions, the answers given can be compared with the Answer Key.
- Extension activities for this lesson could be:
    - Showing the participants various video clips of gross, body humor pranks (e.g., YouTube videos of people pranking each other with a whoopee cushion, fart machines, fake puke or poop)

Reference

Buijzen, M., & Valkenburg, P. (2004). Developing a typology of humor in audiovisual media. *Media Psychology, 6*, 147-167.

EXERCISE: GROSS PRANKS

Today, we are going to do gross pranks. People will think there is something that is really gross, but then they will realize it is fake. Surprise!

Dog Poop Prank

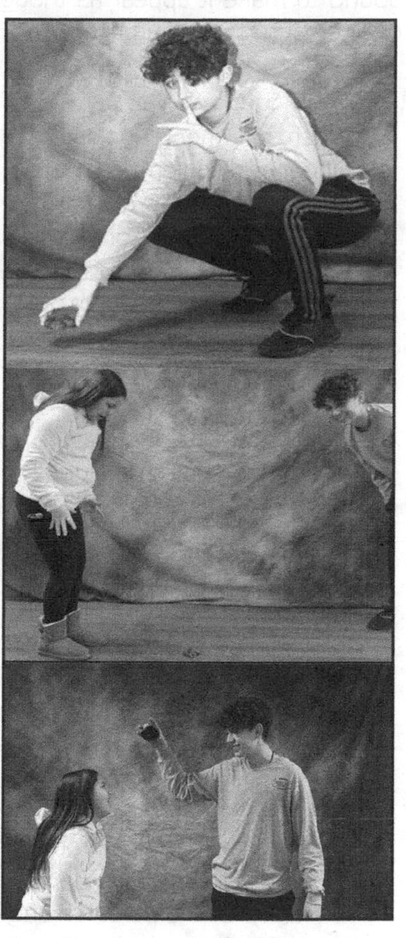

You are going to leave what looks like a dog poop somewhere for someone to find. When someone sees it, he or she will be grossed out. Surprise!

Prank Steps

1. When no one is looking, put the fake dog poop somewhere on the floor where the person can easily see it.
2. When someone comes around, you can say point to the fake poop and say, "Eww! Look what I found!"
3. Watch the person's reaction. Surprise! Then tell the person, "Just kidding! It's fake!"

How Did It Go?

- Did the person smile/laugh?
  Yes No
- Did you smile or laugh?
  Yes No
- Did you think it was funny?
  Yes No

Why Is It Funny?

- Is finding dog poop on the floor inside funny when it is real? No! It is gross and stinky and not nice to clean up.
- When it is just a prank done with the right person at the right time, this can be funny for the person being pranked because it is not what he or she expected to see on the floor.
- It can be funny for the prankster to watch the reaction of the person being pranked, as he or she may jump back and make a funny face.

Whoopee Cushion Prank

You are going to hide a whoopee cushion and get a person to sit on it. When the person sits, it will make a loud sound to make it appear as though he or she passed gas. Surprise!

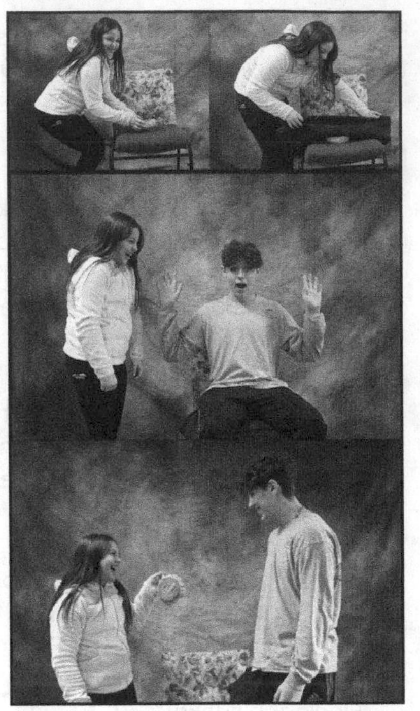

Prank Steps

1. When no one is looking, put the whoopee cushion down on a chair and cover it with a blanket.
2. Ask someone to "Come sit down!"
3. When the person sits down, the whoopee cushion will make a loud sound to make it seem like he or she passed gas! Surprise!

How Did It Go?

- Did the person smile/laugh?
  Yes No
- Did you smile or laugh?
  Yes No
- Did you think it was funny?
  Yes No

Why Is It Funny?

- Is passing gas in front of people always funny? No! While passing gas can be funny because it is a silly sound and a foul smell, if someone is really doing it in front of others, it can be more annoying or gross than funny. It is better to pass gas in the bathroom or away from other people.
- When it is just a prank done with the right person at the right time, this can be funny for the person being pranked because it is not what he or she expected to hear when sitting down.
- It can be funny for the prankster to watch the reaction of the person being pranked, as he or she may jump back and make a funny face!

REVIEW QUESTIONS: GROSS PRANKS

Name:______________________________

1. Is it really funny when a dog poops in the house?
   A. Yes
   B. No
   C. Always

2. Whoopee cushions are funny to use because they:
   A. Make a funny fart noise
   B. Are red
   C. Are small

3. Is it always funny to pass gas in front of people?
   A. Yes
   B. No

4. When you are setting up both gross pranks, you should do it while ______ is looking.
   A. He/she
   B. Everyone
   C. No one

5. It is funny for the prankster to watch the person's ___________ to the prank.
   A. Reaction
   B. Idea
   C. Hands clap

Gross Pranks Review Questions Answer Key

1. B
2. A
3. B
4. C
5. A

Lesson 5: Money Pranks

Objectives

The participant may:

- Understand why money pranks are funny
- Understand how a person can use money pranks to be funny and interact with others

Background

These three pranks are slightly more sophisticated, as they require participants to understand the concept and value of money. This makes it more entertaining when you know why people would work hard to pick up a stuck coin or chase a dollar bill. These pranks require "conceptual incongruity," as the money in the pranks is doing something it does not normally do, which also adds to the humorous aspect (Buijzen & Valkenburg, 2004). Two of the pranks also require a more complex, playful teasing interaction, which is characteristic of older children's humor (Buijzen & Valkenburg, 2004).

Materials

- Money Pranks Visual Story
- Review Questions and Answer Key
- Fake dollar bill
- Tape
- Long piece of white string
- Coin
- Glue
- Cardstock paper
- Quarter
- Pencil
- Mirror

Preparation

- Use the book or photocopy and staple together the visual story entitled Money Pranks
- Photocopy Review Questions, one for each participant
- Make the dollar on a string prank by taping a white string to a fake dollar
- Make the stuck coin prank by gluing a coin onto a piece of cardstock paper
- Make the rolling coin prank by rubbing a pencil on the edge of a quarter

Procedure

- Read the visual story to the participants or have them take turns reading each page. When there are questions, be sure to engage the participants and allow them to answer using their specific mode of communication (speech, communication device, sign language, gestures, etc.). For participants who seem to have a good basic understanding of the concepts in this lesson, ask more challenging questions that make the material more relatable, such as, "Have you ever found money on the ground? Did you try to pick it up? Would you do something silly to make money?"
- When introducing the pranks, first show them by modeling the prank with another adult, if possible. The adult being pranked should have an exaggerated reaction (i.e., wide eyes and surprised look, arms up, and say "AHHHHHH!"). Then, the participant can try it with an adult, who should, again, have an exaggerated reaction. If the activity is being done with a group, the participant should then try the prank with a peer.
- Follow up the activity by having each participant answer the Review Questions, providing assistance as needed. After the participant(s) has completed the questions, the answers given can be compared with the Answer Key.
- Extension activities for this lesson could be:
  - Showing the participants various video clips of pranks related to money on the internet

Reference

Buijzen, M., & Valkenburg, P. (2004). Developing a typology of humor in audiovisual media. *Media Psychology*, 6, 147-167.

EXERCISE: MONEY PRANKS

Today, we are going to do pranks that have to do with money. We will trick people to think they can get some money, but then something else happens. Surprise!

Stuck Coin Prank

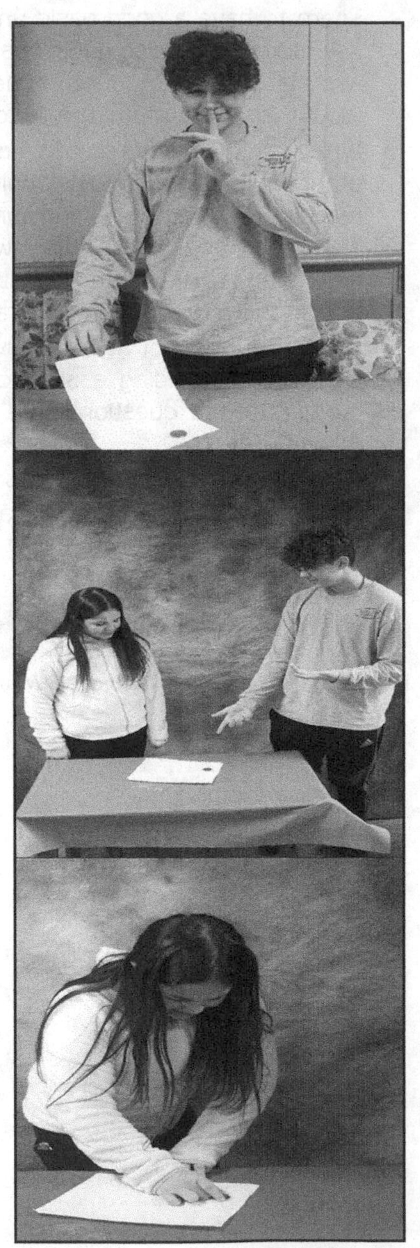

You are going to put down a paper that has a coin stuck to it. When the person goes to pick up the coin, it will be stuck to the paper! Surprise!

Prank Steps

1. When no one is looking, put the paper with the coin stuck to it on a nearby table or the floor.
2. When someone comes around, you can point to the coin and say, "Look, a lucky coin!"
3. Watch as the person tries to pick up the coin, but he or she cannot because it is stuck! Surprise!

How Did It Go?

- Did the person smile/laugh?
  Yes No
- Did you smile or laugh?
  Yes No
- Did you think it was funny?
  Yes No

Why Is It Funny?

- Are coins usually stuck to paper? No! The person being pranked was expecting to just pick up the coin, but it was stuck.
- Because it was not expected that it was stuck, this can be funny for the person being pranked.
- It can be funny to watch someone have a tricky time picking up the stuck coin and can be funny for the person who is trying!

Dollar on a String Prank

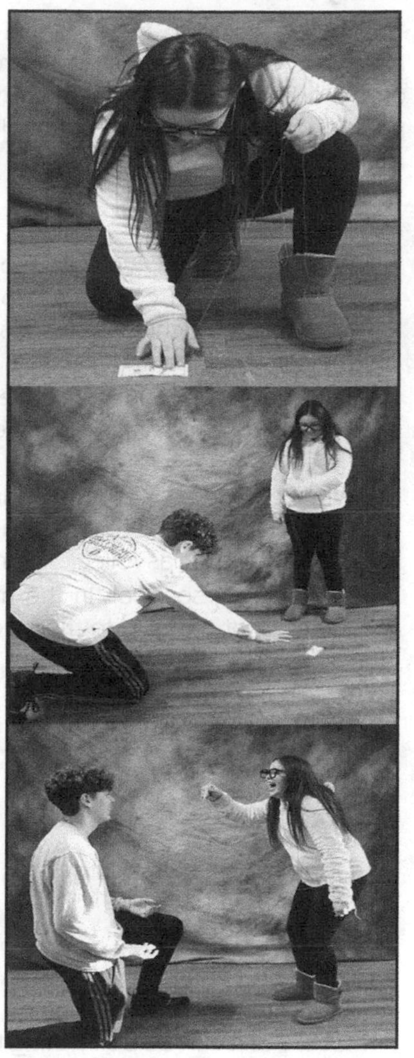

You are going to put a dollar with a string attached to it on the floor and hide. When a person goes to pick up the dollar, you will move the string, and the dollar will move away from the person! Surprise!

Prank Steps

1. When no one is looking, put the dollar with the string attached on the floor.
2. Hold on to the one end of the string and hide.
3. When someone tries to pick up the dollar, pull the string to move the dollar away from him or her. Surprise! The dollar is moving on its own, and the person cannot get the money!

How Did It Go?

- Did the person smile/laugh?
  Yes No
- Did you smile or laugh?
  Yes No
- Did you think it was funny?
  Yes No

Why Is It Funny?

- Do dollar bills usually move away when you try to pick them up? No! Because it was not what he or she expected, this can be funny for the person being pranked.
- It can be funny for the prankster to watch the reaction of the person being pranked and have a tricky time chasing the dollar around!

Rolling Coin Prank

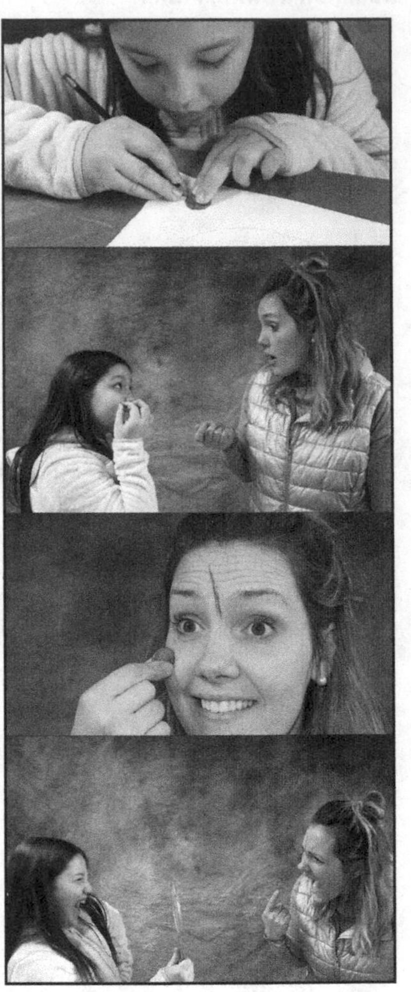

You are going to tell a person that he or she can have a coin if it is rolled on his or her face 10 times. When the person rolls it on his or her face, it will make a mark all over! Surprise!

Prank Steps

1. When no one is looking, rub the outer edge of a coin with a pencil tip. Without touching the edges, put the coin on a table.
2. Tell someone, "You can have my coin if you roll it on your face 10 times."
3. When the person rolls the coin on his or her face, it should make a mark where it was rolled! Surprise!
4. Have the person look in the mirror to see what they did to their face!

How Did It Go?

- Did the person smile/laugh?
  Yes No
- Did you smile or laugh?
  Yes No
- Did you think it was funny?
  Yes No

Why Is It Funny?

- Do people usually roll coins on their face? No! It can be a silly thing to do and to watch someone do, which can be funny for the person being pranked and the prankster.
- Do coins usually leave marks on your face? No! When the person being pranked looks in the mirror, it is funny because it is not what he or she expected. It is funny for the prankster to see the marks on the person's face and to see the person's reaction!

REVIEW QUESTIONS: MONEY PRANKS

Name:________________________________

1. What is the first step of the stuck coin prank?
   A. Put the paper with the stuck coin on a nearby table
   B. Hide
   C. Say, "Look, a lucky coin!"

2. Are coins usually stuck to paper?
   A. No
   B. Yes

3. Do dollar bills normally move away when you try to pick them up?
   A. Yes
   B. No

4. What is one reason the rolling coin prank is funny?
   A. The coin is big
   B. The coin is shiny
   C. The coin leaves marks on a person's face

5. What was your favorite prank today?

Money Pranks Review Questions Answer Key

1. A
2. A
3. B
4. C
5. No wrong answer

CHAPTER 8

Sound and Word Play

Lesson 1: Sound Effects

Objectives

The participant may:

- Learn about the concept of sound effects and what makes them funny
- Understand how a person can make his or her own funny sound effects and use them to interact with others

Background

Before children are able to speak, they imitate words and sounds they hear. When caregivers use silly sounds, such as "raspberries" and high-pitched "weeee" when they move the child around, they are helping to foster good language skills (Children's Hospitals and Clinics of Minnesota, 2013). Later on, children will make sound effects to complement their complex imaginative play, such as making a humming sound for a car motor or various animal sounds when playing with farm toys (Malik & Marwaha, 2019). "Unusual voices and sounds" are often found to be humorous by children when they are first developing their sense of humor, both to hear or to make themselves (Buijzen & Valkenburg, 2004). When children are in Stage 4 of McGhee's humor development, "body sounds" are found to be specifically enjoyable, as they are unexpected, funny sounds that are often taboo to make. This lesson introduces how to make different sounds with your body and demonstrates how the sounds can be used to be funny.

Chaiet, R. *What's So Funny?: Humor-Based Activities for Social Skill Development* (pp. 129-141).

Materials

- Sound Effects Visual Story
- Review Questions and Answer Key
- Sound Effects Story Activity

Preparation

- Use the book or photocopy and staple together the visual story entitled Sound Effects
- Photocopy Review Questions, one for each participant
- Photocopy Sound Effects Story Activity, one copy per participant

Procedure

- Read the visual story to the participants or have them take turns reading each page. When there are questions, be sure to engage the participants and allow them to answer using their specific mode of communication (speech, communication device, sign language, gestures, etc.). For participants who seem to have a good basic understanding of the concepts in this lesson, ask more challenging questions that make the material more relatable, such as, "What sounds do you find funny? What other funny sound can you make using your voice or your body?"
- When introducing the sound effects, first show them by modeling how to make the sound.
- When it is time to do the Sound Effects Story Activity, have the participants make the sound effects as the instructor narrates. If there is more than one participant, the sound effects can be assigned or chosen by the participants.
- Follow up the activity by having each participant answer the Review Questions, providing assistance as needed. After the participant(s) has completed the questions, the answers given can be compared with the Answer Key.
- Extension activities for this lesson could be:
  - Watching performers who make sound effects using their voice or body only or watching an "old time style" radio show that uses a person's voice or objects for sound effects

References

Buijzen, M., & Valkenburg, P. (2004). Developing a typology of humor in audiovisual media. *Media Psychology, 6*, 147-167.

Children's Hospitals and Clinics of Minnesota. (2013). Playing with sounds: Helping young children develop speech skills. *Patient Family Education*. https://www.childrensmn.org/references/pfs/rehab-public/playing-with-sounds.pdf

Malik, F., & Marwaha, R. (2019). *Developmental stages of social emotional development in children*. StatPearls Publishing.

EXERCISE: SOUND EFFECTS

Today, we are going to learn how to make our own sound effects and how to use them to be funny! Have you ever heard a sound that made you laugh? What was it? Funny sounds used in a movie or show are called *sound effects*. Sometimes, people find them funny. Some sound effects can be made with your own body.

You can make "raspberries" or a fart sound by pushing air through your lips against your hand.

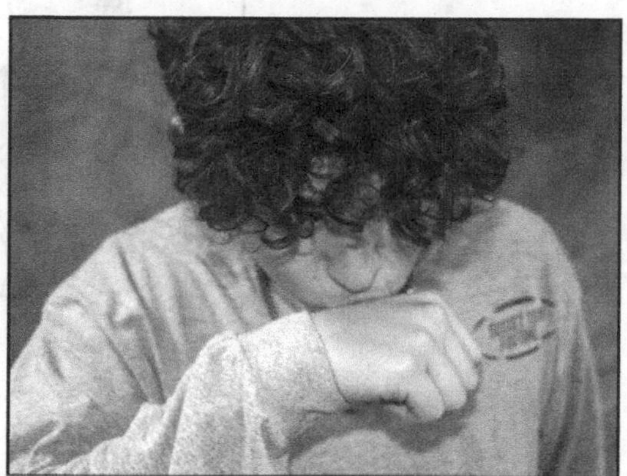

You can make high sounds like:

- A bird tweeting: "TWEET TWEET!"
- A dog whining: "NNNnnnNNnnn!"
- A robot's bee boop: "BEEP BOOP BOP!"

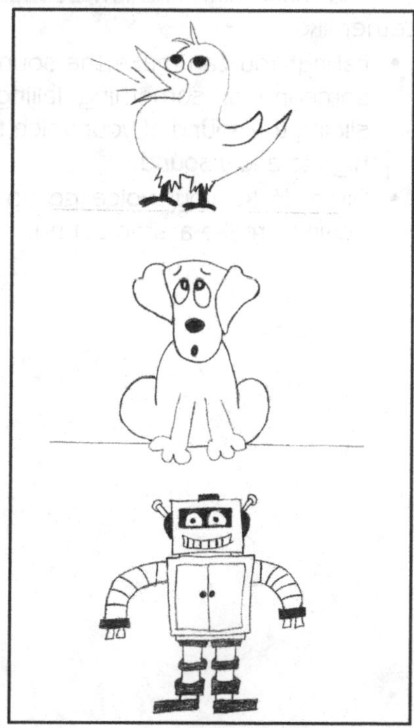

You can make low sounds like:

- A car motor: "RUMBLE!"
- A roaring lion: "ROAR!"
- A fake burp: "UGHH!"

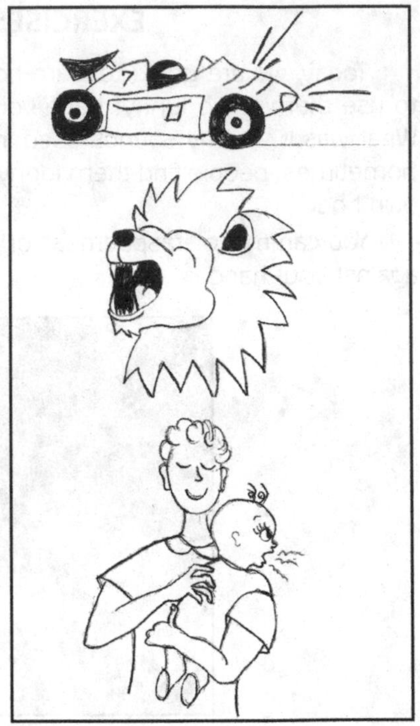

You make high and low sounds together like:

- Falling: You can make the sound of someone or something falling by sliding the sound of your voice from high to a low sound.
- Siren: Make your voice go up and down to make a siren sound.

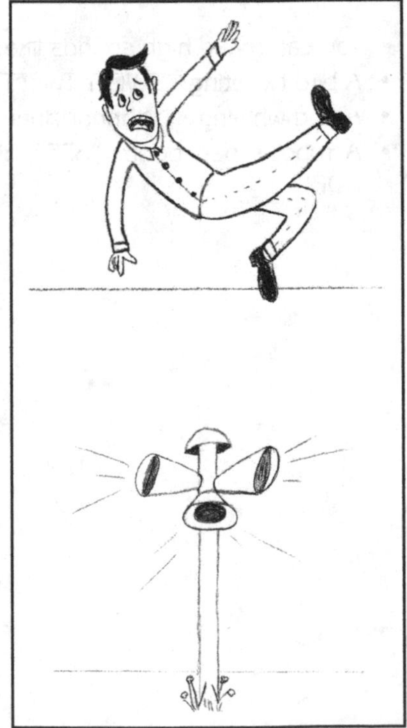

You can also use your hands to help you make sound effects like:

- Car beep: Hold your nose and say "BEEP BEEP!"
- Walking: Move your hands up and down on a table or your lap to make the sound of someone walking.

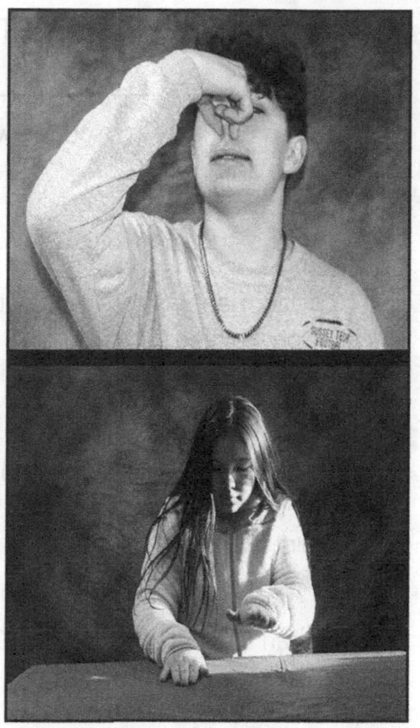

Let's make a funny story using our sound effects!

Have the participant(s) make the sound effects when noted during this crazy story for a good laugh!

Once upon a time there was a ROBOT. (BEEP BOOP BOP sound)

He needed to go to the store, so he WALKED to his car. (WALKING sound)

He started DRIVING to the restaurant. (CAR MOTOR sound)

All of a sudden, he saw a LION in a tree. (ROAR sound). He couldn't believe it!

The robot got out of the car and WALKED over to the tree. (WALKING sound)

Then, the lion FELL out of the tree. (FALLING sound)

It was hurt. Luckily, an AMBULANCE was driving by and stopped to help him. (SIREN sound)

The lion was not moving, and they were worried. But all of a sudden, he let out a big FART. (FART sound)

It was gross, but they were happy the lion was going to be okay.

THE END.

REVIEW QUESTIONS: SOUND EFFECTS

Name: ______________________________

1. You can make funny sounds with what two parts of your body?
   A. Toes and mouth
   B. Hands and mouth
   C. Hands and eyebrows

2. You can make a high-pitch sound to sound like a __________.
   A. Dog whining
   B. Fake burp
   C. Lion roaring

3. You can make a low-pitch sound to sound like a __________.
   A. Robot beep booping
   B. Bird tweeting
   C. Car motor

4. You can make your voice go up and down to sound like a __________.
   A. Giraffe
   B. Siren
   C. Bug

5. When you make a raspberry sound on your hand with your mouth, it is funny because it sounds like a ____________.
   A. Fart
   B. Grass
   C. Cow

Sound Effects Review Questions Answer Key

1. B
2. A
3. C
4. B
5. A

Lesson 2: Rhyming Words

Objectives

The participant may:

- Increase awareness of rhyming words with same ending sounds
- Review words that rhyme and discover how they can be funny to hear, as well as relate to visual incongruities

Background

As children develop, they begin to use words more than actions to express themselves and to engage in playful interactions with others (Semrud-Clikeman & Glass, 2010). Around the age of 8 years, children begin to develop more appreciation for linguistic humor and begin to find basic rhymes and jokes funny (Buijzen & Valkenburg, 2004). According to McGhee, children in Stage 4 of humor development enjoy playing with the sounds of words and playfully distorting aspects of common objects, animals, and people. This lesson introduces funny rhyming words and relates them to humorous visual incongruities, such as "The wee bee went to the tea sea" and others.

Materials

- Rhyming Words Visual Story
- Review Questions and Answer Key

Preparation

- Use the book or photocopy and staple together the visual story entitled Rhyming Words
- Photocopy Review Questions, one for each participant

Procedure

- Read the visual story to the participants or have them take turns reading each page. When there are questions, be sure to engage the participants and allow them to answer using their specific mode of communication (speech, communication device, sign language, gestures, etc.). For participants who seem to have a good basic understanding of the concepts in this lesson, ask more challenging questions that make the material more relatable, such as, "Have you ever heard a funny poem or nursery rhyme? What was it?"
- Follow up the activity by having each participant answer the Review Questions, providing assistance as needed. After the participant(s) has completed the questions, the answers given can be compared with the Answer Key.
- Extension activities for this lesson could be:
  - Reading or listening to Dr. Seuss books or other humorous books with rhyming words

References

Buijzen, M., & Valkenburg, P. (2004). Developing a typology of humor in audiovisual media. *Media Psychology, 6*, 147-167.

Semrud-Clikeman, M., & Glass, K. (2010). The relation of humor and child development: Social, adaptive and emotional aspects. *Journal of Child Neurology, 25*(10), 1248-1260.

EXERCISE: RHYMING WORDS

Today, we are going to talk about words that sound the same and how to use them to be funny! Do you know what words that sound the same are called? They are called *rhyming words*.

For example, cat has an "at" sound. It rhymes with words that also have the "at" sound like:

- Bat
- Fat
- Gnat
- Hat
- Mat
- Rat
- Sat
- Tat

A silly sentence using "at" words could be:
A FAT CAT SAT on a RAT.

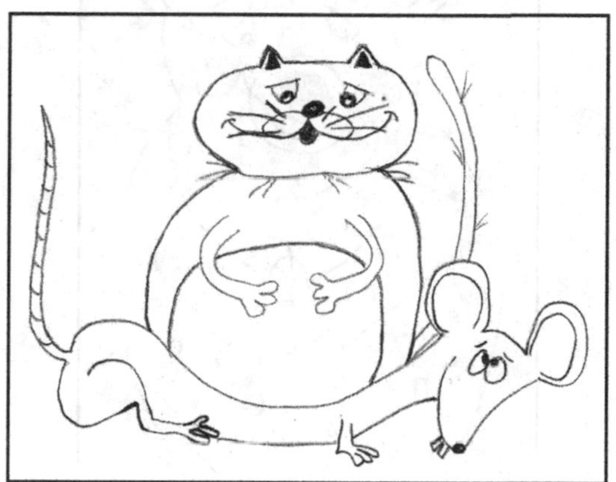

Can you make another silly sentence with "at" sound words?

A ______ ______ sat on a ______.

Bat Fat Gnat Hat Mat Rat Sat Tat

- Does it sound funny?
- Is it funny to think about this happening?

Bear has an "air" sound and rhymes with words that also have the "air" sound, even if the spelling is different, like:

- Air
- Care
- Fair
- Hair
- Pear
- Rare
- Square
- Stare
- Tear
- Where

A silly sentence using these words could be:
A RARE BEAR had a SQUARE PEAR.

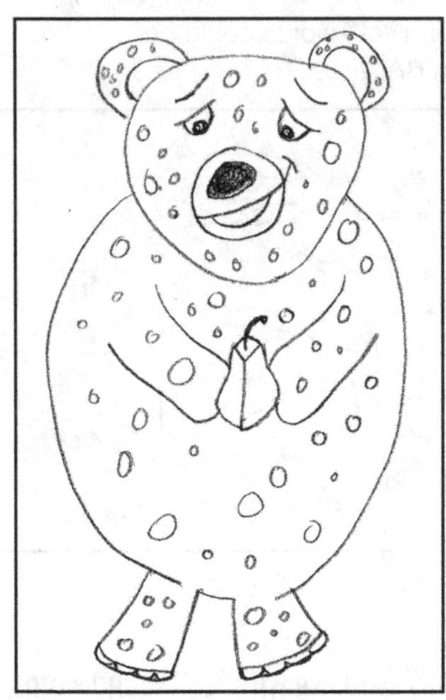

Can you make another silly sentence with the "air" sound words?

A ______ ________ had a ______ _______.

Air Care Fair Hair Pear Rare Square Stare Tear Where

- Does it sound funny?
- Is it funny to think about this happening?

Bee has an "ee" sound and rhymes with words that also have the "ee" sound, even if the spelling is different, like:

- Fee
- Key
- Knee
- Me
- Pea
- Sea
- Tea
- Tree
- Wee

A silly sentence using these words could be:
The WEE BEE went to the TEA SEA.

Can you make another silly sentence with the "ee" sound words?

The ______ ______ went to the ______ ______.

Fee Key Knee Me Pea Sea Tea Tree Wee

- Does it sound funny?
- Is it funny to think about this happening?

Some silly sayings also have rhyming words in them.
For example, "See you later, Alligator!"
Later and Alligator have the "ater" sound.

Can you figure out the rest of the sayings by finding the rhyming word?

After a while, ____________________.
Give me a hug, ____________________.
See you soon, ____________________.
Hit the road, ____________________.
Open the door, ____________________.

Crocodile Dinosaur Ladybug Raccoon Toad

REVIEW QUESTIONS: RHYMING WORDS

Name:______________________________

1. Words that rhyme have the same ______________.
   A. First letter
   B. Look
   C. Sound

2. What word rhymes with bug?
   A. Rug
   B. Boo
   C. Dog

3. What word rhymes with car?
   A. Cool
   B. Far
   C. Cat

4. What word rhymes with toe?
   A. Finger
   B. Slow
   C. Hand

5. What silly saying did you like best?
   A. After a while, crocodile.
   B. See you soon, raccoon.
   C. Open the door, dinosaur.

Rhyming Words Review Questions Answer Key

1. C
2. A
3. B
4. B
5. No wrong answer

CHAPTER 9

Jokes

Lesson 1: Rhyming Jokes

Objectives

The participant may:

- Increase awareness of question-and-answer jokes with rhymes in them
- Understand why rhyming jokes are funny
- Understand how a person can use rhyming question-and-answer jokes to be funny and interact with peers

Background

As children become more fluent in their ability to use language to communicate and socialize, they are better able to use language in more clever ways. In Stage 5 of McGhee's humor development, children begin to have a better understanding of how words can have multiple meanings and begin to effectively use riddles and jokes (Cunningham, 2004). The first jokes that are appreciated by children are those that are related to the phoneme, including jokes with rhyming words as part of the punchline (Schumann, 2008). This lesson introduces various rhyming jokes, relates them to humorous visual incongruities, and encourages the participants to practice saying these jokes.

Materials

- Rhyming Jokes Visual Story
- Review Questions and Answer Key

Preparation

- Use the book or photocopy and staple together the visual story entitled Rhyming Jokes
- Photocopy Review Questions, one for each participant

Procedure

- Read the visual story to the participants or have them take turns reading each page. When there are questions, be sure to engage the participants and allow them to answer using their specific mode of communication (speech, communication device, sign language, gestures, etc.). For participants who seem to have a good basic understanding of the concepts in this lesson, ask more challenging questions that make the material more relatable, such as, "Have you ever heard a funny joke with rhyming words? What was it?"
- Follow up the activity by having each participant answer the Review Questions, providing assistance as needed. After the participant(s) has completed the questions, the answers given can be compared with the Answer Key.
- Extension activities for this lesson could be:
  - Reading or listening to additional rhyming question-and-answer jokes and reviewing for each what rhymes and what makes the joke funny

References

Cunningham, J. (2004). Children's humor. In W. G. Scarlett (Ed.), *Children's play* (pp. 93-109). Sage Publications, Inc.

Schumann, N. V. (2008, April). *What's so funny? The auditory and verbal skills of humor*. Presented at the New Jersey Speech-Language-Hearing Association 2008 Annual Convention, Atlantic City, NJ.

EXERCISE: RHYMING JOKES

We talked about funny words that rhyme. Today, we are going to talk about jokes that use rhyming words and how to use them to be funny!

What Is a Joke?

Jokes are a group of words a person says to be funny and make people laugh. First, we will learn about question-and-answer jokes.

Question-and-Answer Jokes

In question-and-answer jokes, you ask a silly question and then give a silly answer. Rhyming question-and-answer jokes give a silly answer that rhymes with a more realistic answer.

Let's start with this one:

Question: Why did the banana go to the doctor?
Answer: He was PEELING bad.

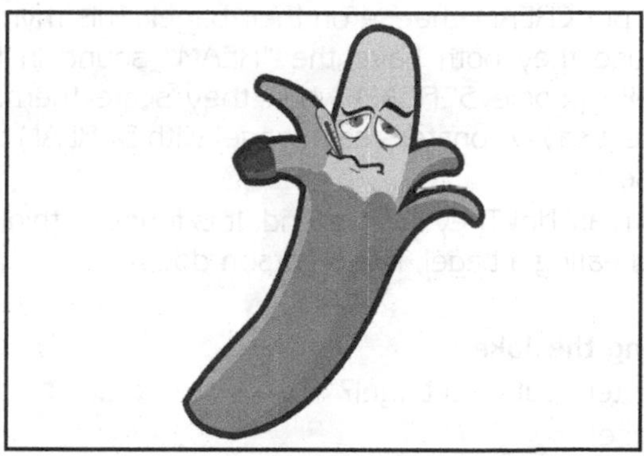

Why Is This Joke Funny?

- People go to the doctor when they are FEELING bad. This rhymes with PEELING, as they both have "EELING" in them. Peeling is what you do to a banana to eat it. This joke is funny because it says the banana is PEELING bad instead of FEELING bad.
- Wait—do bananas go to the doctor? No! A banana is a fruit. Only people go to the doctor. It is funny to think of a banana visiting a doctor because it is not alive and does not get sick like a person.

Practice Saying the Joke

Why did the banana go to the doctor?
He was PEELING bad.

Here's another one:

Question: What do monsters put on a bagel?
Answer: SCREAM cheese!

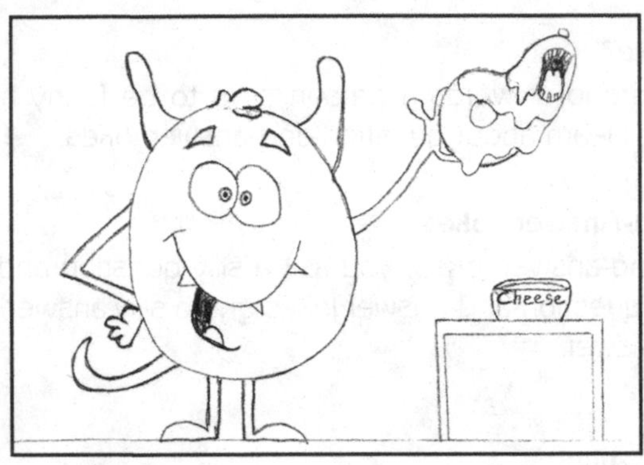

Why Is This Joke Funny?

- Some people put CREAM cheese on their bagel. This rhymes with SCREAM cheese because they both have the "REAM" sound in them. In stories, monsters make people SCREAM when they scare them. So, this joke is funny because it says monsters eat a bagel with SCREAM cheese instead of CREAM cheese.
- Are monsters real? No! They are pretend. It is funny to think about monsters being real and eating a bagel, like a person does.

Practice Saying the Joke

What do monsters put on a bagel?
SCREAM cheese!

Here's another one:

Question: What do birds give out on Halloween?
Answer: TWEETS!

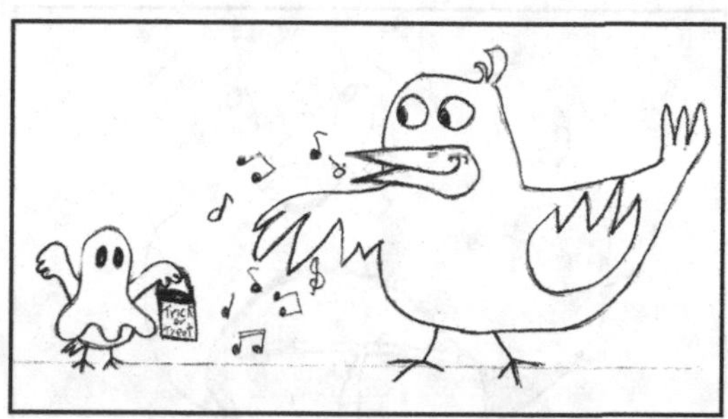

Why Is This Joke Funny?

- On Halloween, we give out TREATS. This rhymes with TWEET because they both have the "EAT" sound in them. TWEET is the sound a bird makes. So, this joke is funny because it says birds give out TWEETS instead of TREATS.
- Do birds give out candy on Halloween? No! They are animals! People give out candy. It is funny to think about birds giving out candy to trick-or-treaters like a person!

Practice Saying the Joke

What do birds give out on Halloween?
TWEETS!

Next joke:

Question: What do clouds wear?
Answer: THUNDERWEAR!

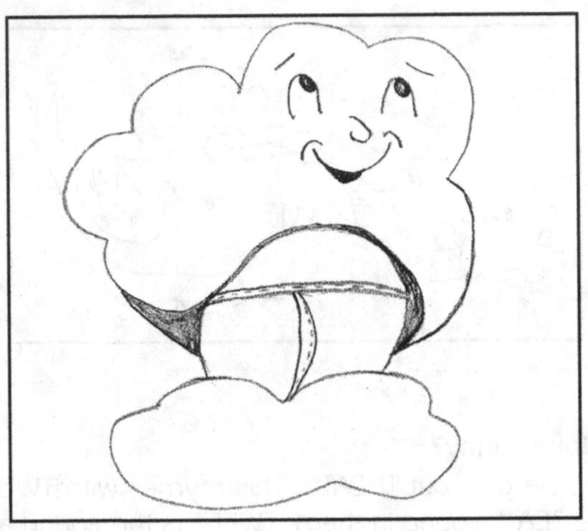

Why Is This Joke Funny?

- People wear UNDERWEAR under their clothes. This rhymes with THUNDERWEAR because they both have the "UNDER" sound in them. When it is cloudy and rainy, sometimes there is THUNDER. So, this joke is funny because it says clouds wear THUNDERWEAR.
- Do clouds wear clothes? No! They are not people! It is funny to think about clouds wearing clothes like a person.

Practice Saying the Joke

What do clouds wear?
THUNDERWEAR!

REVIEW QUESTIONS: RHYMING JOKES

Name:______________________________

1. ______ are a group of words a person says to be funny and make people laugh.
   A. Tricks
   B. Jokes
   C. Nouns

2. In this joke, what word is the rhyming word "glow" replacing to make it funny?
   Question: What did the firefly say to her sister when she won the race?
   Answer: You GLOW girl!
   A. Go
   B. Yo
   C. Cool

3. What else makes the joke funny?
   A. Fireflies fly
   B. Fireflies are small
   C. Fireflies don't talk!

4. When you tell question-and-answer jokes, you ask a silly question and then give a silly __________ .
   A. Answer
   B. Lie
   C. Laugh

5. What was your favorite joke today?

Rhyming Jokes Review Questions Answer Key

1. B
2. A
3. C
4. A
5. No wrong answer

Lesson 2: Homophone Jokes

Objectives

The participant may:

- Increase awareness of question-and-answer jokes with homophones in them
- Understand why homophone jokes are funny
- Understand how a person can use homophone question-and-answer jokes to be funny and interact with peers

Background

Between the ages of 6 to 8 years, typical-developing children begin to understand more complexities in language, such as words like "cool" having more than one meaning (Levine & Munsch, 2010). This newfound skill can be applied to their developing sense of humor. They begin to be able to use homophone jokes, which are those in which the punchline uses a word that sounds like something else to make it funny (Schumann, 2008). These types of jokes are often more challenging for individuals with intellectual disabilities. However, research has shown that by practicing how to decode word meanings, they can improve their ability to understand and use homophone jokes (Agius & Levey, 2019). This lesson introduces various homophone jokes, relates them to humorous visual incongruities, and encourages the participants to practice saying these jokes.

Materials

- Homophone Jokes Visual Story
- Review Questions and Answer Key

Preparation

- Use the book or photocopy and staple together the visual story entitled Homophone Jokes
- Photocopy Review Questions, one for each participant

Procedure

- Read the visual story to the participants or have them take turns reading each page. When there are questions, be sure to engage the participants and allow them to answer using their specific mode of communication (speech, communication device, sign language, gestures, etc.). For participants who seem to have a good basic understanding of the concepts in this lesson, ask more challenging questions that make the material more relatable, such as, "Have you ever heard of puns? Do you know any words that have two meanings?"
- Follow up the activity by having each participant answer the Review Questions, providing assistance as needed. After the participant(s) has completed the questions, the answers given can be compared with the Answer Key.
- Extension activities for this lesson could be:
    - Reading or listening to additional homophone question-and-answer jokes and reviewing for each what sounds alike and what makes the joke funny.

References

Agius, J., & Levey, S. (2019). Humor intervention approaches for children, adolescents and adults. *Israeli Journal for Humor Research, 8*(1), 8-28.

Levine, L., & Munsch, J. (2010). *Child development: An active learning approach.* Sage Publications, Inc.

Schumann, N. V. (2008, April). *What's so funny? The auditory and verbal skills of humor.* Presented at the New Jersey Speech-Language-Hearing Association 2008 Annual Convention, Atlantic City, NJ.

EXERCISE: HOMOPHONE JOKES

Today, we are going to learn more jokes. This time, we will talk about question-and-answer jokes that use homophones and how to use them to be funny! Homophones are words that sound like other words but mean something different. They are funny in jokes because silly words are used that sound like the more realistic word.

Let's start with this one:

Question: How does a chicken stay healthy?

Answer: EGGs-ercise!

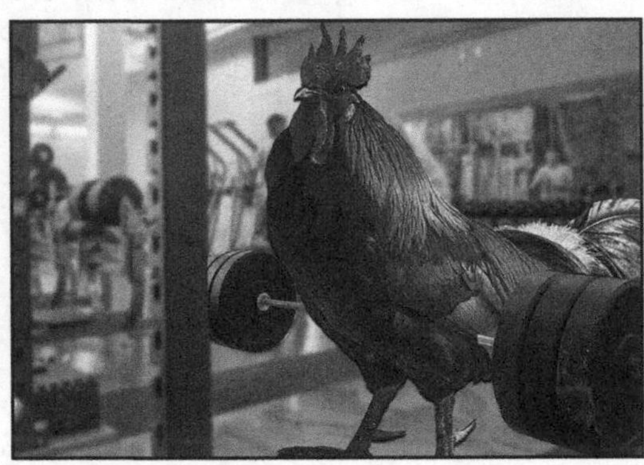

Why Is This Joke Funny?

- EGGs-ercise sounds like EX-ercise. EGG was put in the word because chickens lay eggs. It is funny to put EGG into the word EX-ercise to describe how chickens stay healthy.
- Do chickens exercise? No! People exercise to stay healthy. It is funny to think of chickens lifting weights or running on a treadmill like a person!

Practice Saying the Joke

How does a chicken stay healthy?

EGGs-ercise!

Here's another one:

Question: How did the ghost look in her dress?
Answer: BOO-tiful!

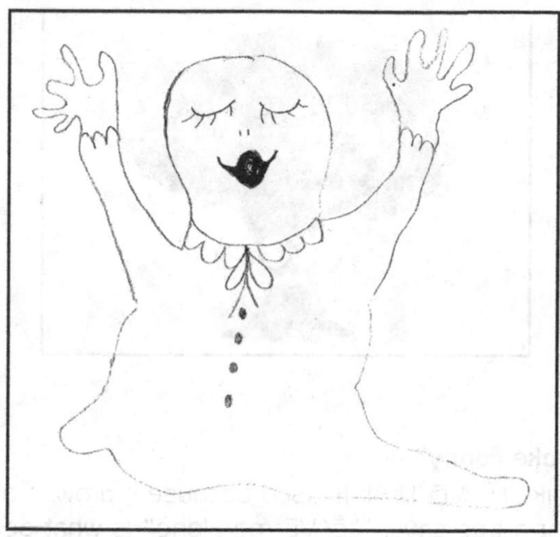

Why Is This Joke Funny?

- BOO-tiful sounds like BEAU-tiful. "BOO" is used because it is what ghosts say in scary stories. It is funny to put that into the word BEAU-tiful to describe a ghost's dress.
- Are ghosts real? No! When ghosts are in stories, they are usually scary and do not wear beautiful dresses, either! So, it is funny to think of ghosts wearing beautiful dresses like a person does.

Practice Saying the Joke

How did the ghost look in her dress?
BOO-tiful!

Here's another one:

Question: What did the tree say when he was cranky?
Answer: LEAF me alone!

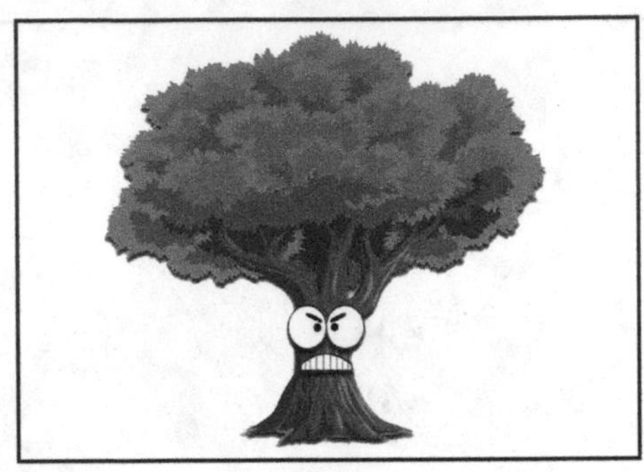

Why Is This Joke Funny?

- LEAF sounds like LEAVE. LEAF is used because it grows from a tree and the joke asks what a tree says. "LEAVE me alone" is what people might say if they are cranky. So, it is funny to use LEAF instead of the word LEAVE.
- Do trees get cranky or have other emotions? No! People do! Do trees talk? No! People do! It is funny to think of trees having feelings and talking about it like a person.

Practice Saying the Joke

What did the tree say when he was cranky?
LEAF me alone!

Here's another one:

Question: What kind of flower grows on your face?
Answer: TWO-lips!

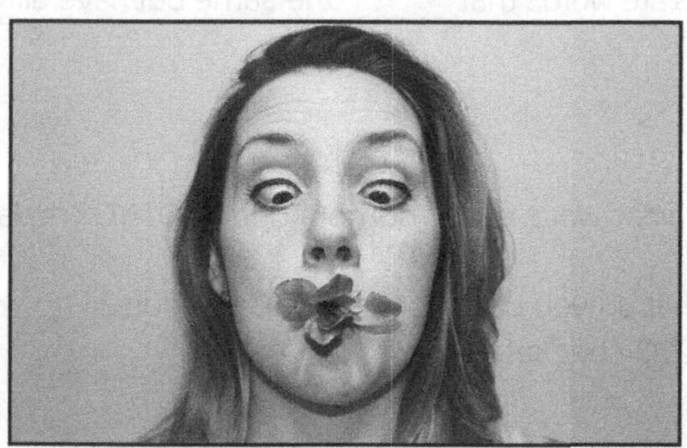

Why Is This Joke Funny?

- TWO-lips sounds like TU-lips. TULIPS are a type of flower. People have TWO lips on their face. It is funny to use TWO-lips instead of TULIPS.
- Do people grow flowers on their face? No! Flowers grow out of the ground. It is silly to think of flowers growing out of your face!

Practice Saying the Joke

Question: What kind of flower grows on your face?
Answer: TWO-lips!

REVIEW QUESTIONS: HOMOPHONE JOKES

Name: ______________________________

1. Homophones are words that ______ the same but have different meanings.
   A. Look
   B. Sound
   C. Smell

2. In this joke, what word is the homophone "NOT-YO" replacing to make it funny?
   Question: What do you call cheese that isn't yours?
   Answer: NOT-YO cheese!
   A. Nacho
   B. Gouda
   C. Cheddar

3. In this joke, besides the homophone, what makes it funny?
   Question: What kind of flower grows on your face?
   Answer: TWO-lips!
   A. Tulips smell
   B. Flowers do not grow on your face
   C. People do not have lips

4. Why do we tell jokes?
   A. To be funny
   B. To be mean
   C. To be sad

5. What was your favorite joke today?

Homophone Jokes Review Questions Answer Key

1. B
2. A
3. B
4. A
5. No wrong answer

Lesson 3: Silly Sound Jokes

Objectives

The participant may:

- Increase awareness of question-and-answer jokes with silly sounds in them
- Understand why silly sound jokes are funny
- Use physical comedy gestures to improve ability to understand and tell the jokes
- Understand how a person can use silly sound jokes to be funny and interact with peers

Background

The jokes in this lesson are very similar to those in the previous, as they continue to use homophones. However, the "same sound word" that is used in each joke is a "silly sound" that an animal, person, or object makes. In addition, the participant is encouraged to act out the animal, person, or thing making that sound during the punchline of the joke using the techniques learned in the previous Funny Faces and Impressions lessons. For some, these jokes may be even more enjoyable, as one study showed that using physical gestures while telling jokes helps individuals with intellectual disabilities to understand them better (Degabriele & Walsh, 2010). This lesson introduces various silly sound jokes and encourages the participants to use funny facial expressions and body movements when they tell them to others.

Materials

- Silly Sound Jokes Visual Story
- Review Questions and Answer Key
- Mirror

Preparation

- Use the book or photocopy and staple together the visual story entitled Silly Sound Jokes
- Photocopy Review Questions, one for each participant

Procedure

- Read the visual story to the participants or have them take turns reading each page. When there are questions, be sure to engage the participants and allow them to answer using their specific mode of communication (speech, communication device, sign language, gestures, etc.). For participants who seem to have a good basic understanding of the concepts in this lesson, ask more challenging questions that make the material more relatable, such as "Have you ever heard of a joke with a silly sound in it? Do you remember the funny faces we talked about in another lesson? Do you remember the impressions we talked about in another lesson?"
- Follow up the activity by having each participant answer the Review Questions, providing assistance as needed. After the participant(s) has completed the questions, the answers given can be compared with the Answer Key.
- Extension activities for this lesson could be:
    - Reading or listening to additional silly sound question-and-answer jokes and reviewing for each what word the silly sounds sound like and what makes the joke funny

Reference

Degabriele, J., & Walsh, I. (2010). Humour appreciation and comprehension in children with intellectual disability. *Journal of Intellectual Disability Research, 54*(6), 525-538.

EXERCISE: SILLY SOUND JOKES

Today, we are going to learn about jokes that use silly sounds. We will use animal noises and other sounds to make the joke funny! Remember the slapstick and impression lessons? In these jokes, we will use big facial expressions and big movements to make the joke even funnier!

Let's start with this one:

Question: Where did the cow go on Friday?
Answer: To the MOOOOvies.

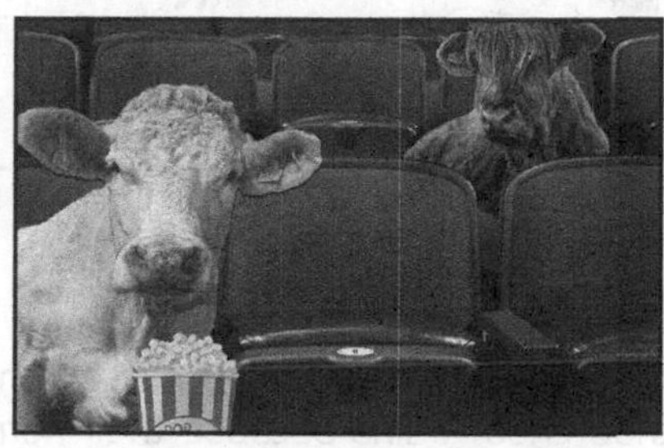

Why Is This Joke Funny?

- MOOOO is the sound a cow makes. The word movies starts with the "moo" sound. So, it is funny to say when a cow goes to the movies, he goes to the MOOOOvies.
- Wait—do cows go to the movies? No! People do. It is funny to think of a cow walking into a movie theater and sitting down to eat popcorn and watch a movie like a person!

Big Faces and Movements

When you say MOOOOvies, you are going to do an impression of a cow.

- Big cow lips
- Lift your head up like a cow

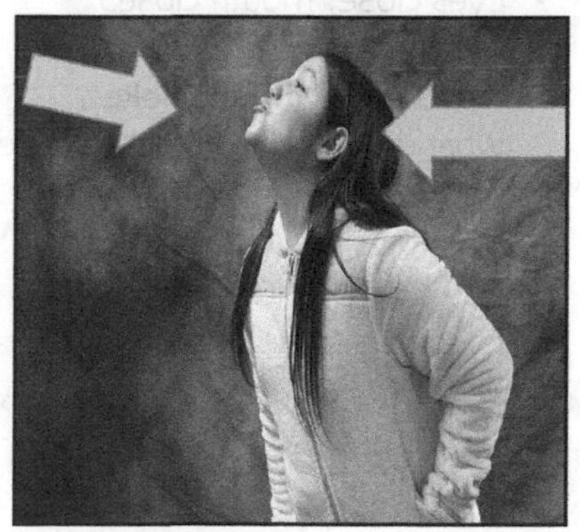

Practice Saying the Joke

Say: Where did the cow go on Friday?

Big cow lips, lift your head up like a cow

Say: To the MOOOOvies!

Here's another one:

Question: What do you call a train that sneezes?
Answer: AAAA-CHOO CHOO train!

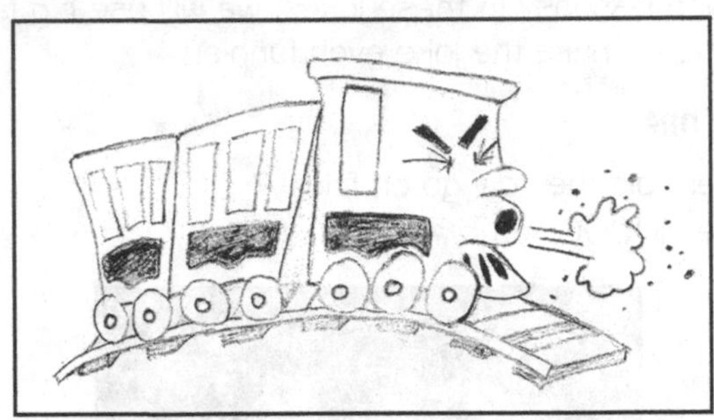

Why Is This Joke Funny?

- The "AAAA-CHOO!" sound is made when a person sneezes. People sometimes call trains "choo choo" trains because their horns can make a "choo choo" sound. So, it is funny to say a train says "AAAA-CHOO CHOO" when it sneezes.
- Wait—do trains sneeze? No! People do! It is funny to think of a train that is sick and sneezing like a person does.

Big Faces and Movements

When you say AAAA-CHOO CHOO train, you are going to do a big sneeze face.

- Eyebrows down, mouth open
- Eyes close, mouth closes

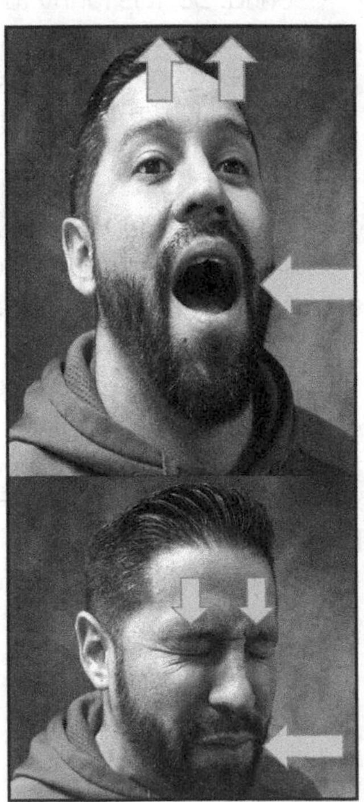

Practice Saying the Joke

What do you call a train that sneezes?
Say: AAAA-
Eyebrows down, mouth open
Say: CHOO CHOO train!
Eyebrows close, mouth closes

Here's another one:

Question: What do you call a horse that lives next door?
Answer: Your NEIGHHH-bor!

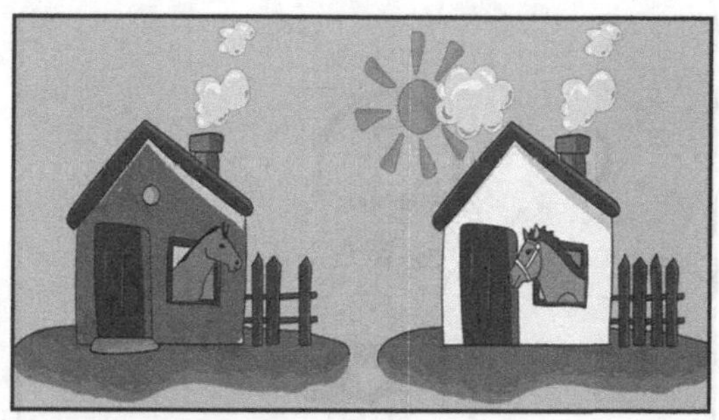

Why Is This Joke Funny?

- NEIGHHH is the sound a horse makes. The word neighbor starts with the "neigh" sound. So, it is funny to say a horse that lives next door is your NEIGHHH-bor.
- Wait—are horses your neighbors? No! People are. It is funny to think of a horse living in the house next to you and being your neighbor like a person is.

Big Faces and Movements

When you say NEIGHHH-bor, you are going to do an impression of a horse.

- Lift your head up like a horse
- Shake your head back and forth like a horse
- Say: NEIGHHH-bor!

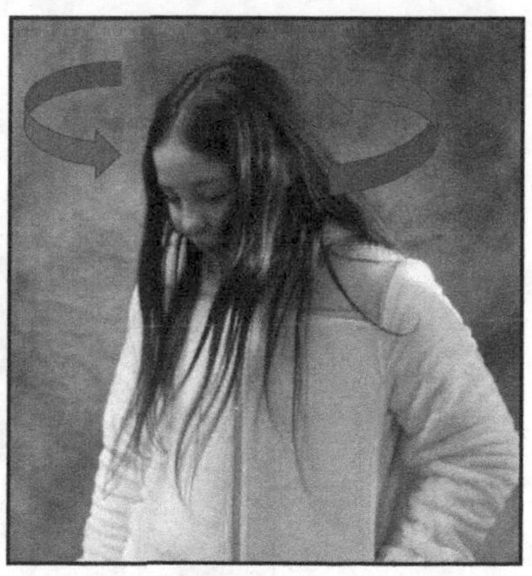

Practice Saying the Joke

Say: What do you call a horse that lives next door?

Lift your head up like a horse

Shake your head back and forth like a horse

Say: Your NEIGHHH-bor!

Here's another one:

Question: Why are pirates called pirates?
Answer: Because they ARRRRRR.

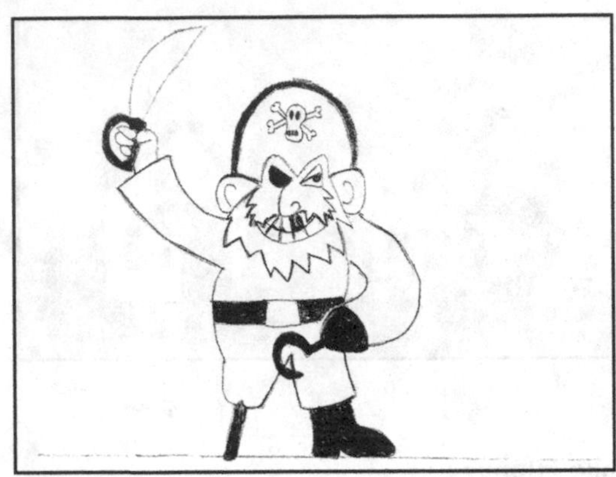

Why Is This Joke Funny?

- ARRRRRR is the sound a pirate makes in stories. Because the question is about pirates, it is funny to say "ARRRRRR" instead of "are" because they have the same sound.

Big Faces and Movements

When you say ARRRRRR, you are going to do an impression of a pirate.

- Make a hook with your pointer finger
- Angry pirate face

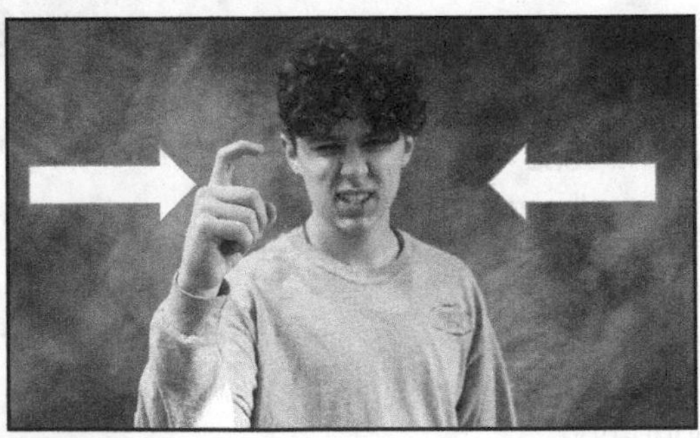

Practice Saying the Joke

Say: Why are pirates called pirates?
Make a hook with your pointer finger
Angry pirate face
Say: Because they ARRRRRR.

REVIEW QUESTIONS: SILLY SOUND JOKES

Name: ____________________________

1. In silly sound jokes, we can use big facial expressions and big ________ to make the joke even funnier.
   A. Movements
   B. Hats
   C. Ears

2. Why is PURRRR-ple a funny answer in this joke?
   Question: What is a cat's favorite color?
   Answer: PURRRR-ple!
   A. Purple is a dark color
   B. Purple starts with P
   C. Purple starts with a cat's "PURRRR" sound

3. What else makes this joke funny?
   A. Cats do not have a favorite color
   B. Cats meow
   C. Purple is not a color

4. What movement could you add to the cat joke to make it funnier?
   A. Do a frog jump
   B. Pretend to lick your paws
   C. Slither like a snake

5. What was your favorite joke today?

Silly Sound Jokes Review Questions Answer Key

1. A
2. C
3. A
4. B
5. No wrong answer

Lesson 4: Knock-Knock Jokes

Objectives

The participant may:

- Increase understanding of knock-knock jokes
- Understand why knock-knock jokes are funny
- Understand how a person can use knock-knock jokes to be funny and interact with peers

Background

This final joke lesson highlights a favorite: knock-knock jokes. The ones used in this lesson require the same type of humor comprehension as previous lessons, as they use either homophones or silly sounds. However, the format of the jokes is different. Knock-knock jokes require a dialogue between two people instead of just one person asking a question and giving a funny answer. This back and forth always uses the same structure, with the joke teller always saying, "Knock-knock" and the recipient of the joke always saying the same, "Who's there?" and "______, who?". Because it is so structured, a visual script can be used, which is a list of words or pictorial examples that assists individuals with socialization challenges engage in social exchanges (Ganz, 2007). This lesson introduces various knock-knock jokes, relates them to humorous visual incongruities, and encourages the participants to practice saying these jokes using a visual script, if needed.

Materials

- Knock-Knock Jokes Visual Story
- Review Questions and Answer Key

Preparation

- Use the book or photocopy and staple together the visual story entitled Knock-Knock Jokes
- Photocopy Review Questions, one for each participant

Procedure

- Read the visual story to the participants or have them take turns reading each page. When there are questions, be sure to engage the participants and allow them to answer using their specific mode of communication (speech, communication device, sign language, gestures, etc.). For participants who seem to have a good basic understanding of the concepts in this lesson, ask more challenging questions that make the material more relatable, such as "Have you ever heard a knock-knock joke? Do you remember how to tell it?"
- Follow up the activity by having each participant answer the Review Questions, providing assistance as needed. After the participant(s) has completed the questions, the answers given can be compared with the Answer Key.
- Extension activities for this lesson could be:
  - Reading or listening to knock-knock jokes and reviewing what word the silly sounds sound like and what makes the joke funny.

Reference

Ganz, J. B. (2007). Classroom structuring methods and strategies for children and youth with autism spectrum disorders. *Exceptionality, 15*, 249-260.

EXERCISE: KNOCK-KNOCK JOKES

Today, we will learn a new type of joke: a "knock-knock" joke. This type of joke takes two people to tell. One person pretends he or she is knocking at a door and says, "Knock-knock." The other person pretends to answer the door and says, "Who's there?" They go back and forth once again, and then the first person ends with the funny ending or punchline. The punchline usually uses a homophone, like some of the question-and-answer jokes we learned about.

Let's start with this one:

Person 1: Knock knock.
Person 2: Who's there?
Person 1: Doughnut.
Person 2: Doughnut, who?
Person 1: DOUGH NOT ask! Open the door!

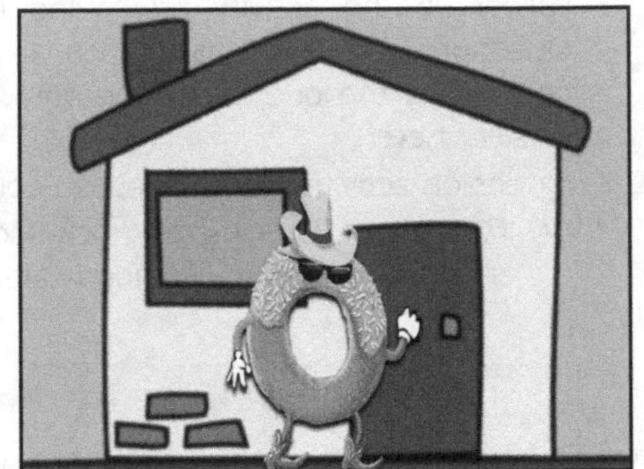

Why Is This Joke Funny?

- Doughnut, which is a dessert food, sounds like DO NOT. So, doughnut is used in place of "do not" to be funny in the sentence "DOUGH NOT ask!"
- Do doughnuts knock on doors? No! They do not have arms and hands, and they do not move on their own. It is funny to think of a doughnut knocking on a door like a person!
- Do doughnuts talk? No! It is funny to think of a doughnut having a mouth and talking like a person.

Practice Saying the Joke

Person 1: Knock knock.
Person 2: Who's there?
Person 1: Doughnut.
Person 2: Doughnut, who?
Person 1: DOUGH NOT ask! Open the door!

Here's another one:

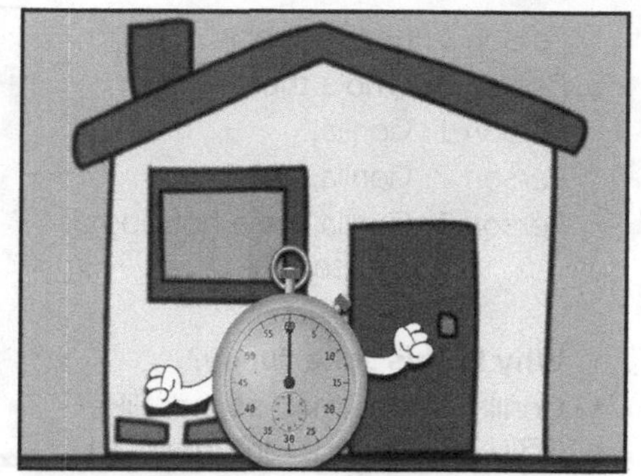

Person 1: Knock knock.
Person 2: Who's there?
Person 1: Stopwatch.
Person 2: Stopwatch, who?
Person 1: Stopwatch you are doing and open the door!

Why Is This Joke Funny?

- Stopwatch, a type of watch, sounds like STOP WHAT. So, stopwatch is used in place of it "stop what" to be funny in the sentence "Stopwatch you are doing."
- Do stopwatches knock on doors? No! They do not have arms and hands and they do not move on their own. It is funny to think of a stopwatch knocking on a door like a person!
- Do stopwatches talk? No! It is funny to think of a stopwatch having a mouth and talking like a person.

Practice Saying the Joke

Person 1: Knock knock.
Person 2: Who's there?
Person 1: Stopwatch.
Person 2: Stopwatch, who?
Person 1: Stopwatch you are doing and open the door!

Here's another one:

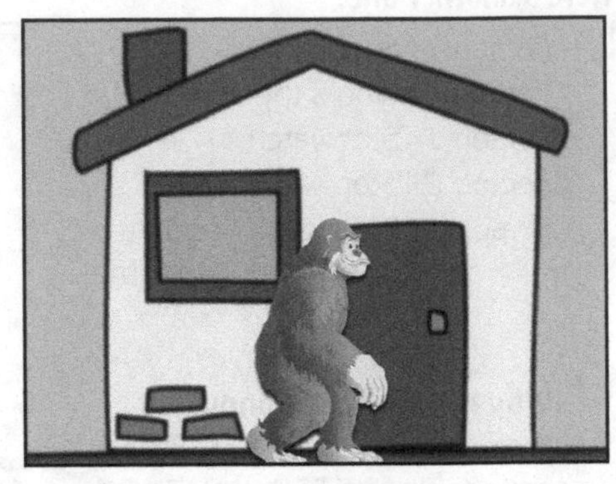

Person 1: Knock knock.
Person 2: Who's there?
Person 1: Gorilla.
Person 2: Gorilla, who?
Person 1: Gorilla me a hot dog, please!

Why Is This Joke Funny?

- Gorilla, the animal, sounds like GRILL A, as in a grill used to cook food. So, gorilla is used in place of "grill a" to be funny in the sentence, "Gorilla me a hot dog, please."

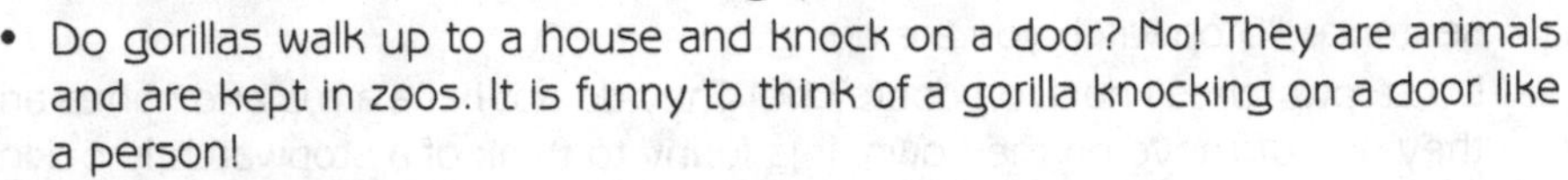

- Do gorillas walk up to a house and knock on a door? No! They are animals and are kept in zoos. It is funny to think of a gorilla knocking on a door like a person!
- Do gorillas talk? No! It is funny to think of a gorilla talking and asking for a hot dog like a person.
- When you knock on someone's door, do you ask him or her to make you some food? No! It is funny to think of someone knocking on a person's door and asking them for a hot dog. How rude!

Practice Saying the Joke

Person 1: Knock knock.
Person 2: Who's there?
Person 1: Gorilla.
Person 2: Gorilla, who?
Person 1: Gorilla me a hot dog, please!

Here's another one:

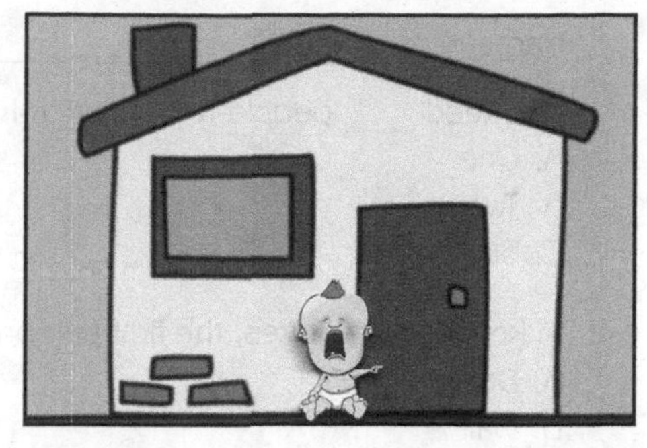

Person 1: Knock knock.
Person 2: Who's there?
Person 1: Boo.
Person 2: Boo, who?
Person 1: Don't cry! It's only a joke.

Why Is This Joke Funny?

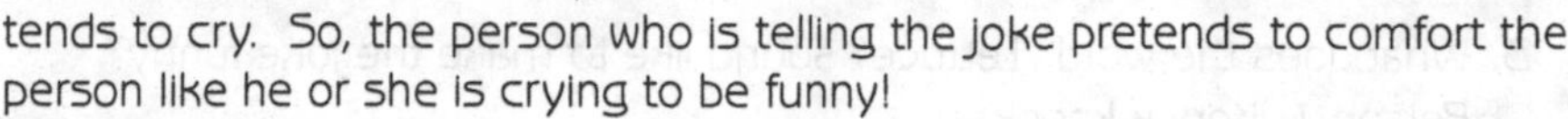

- "Boo, who?" sounds like BOO-HOO, the sound a person makes when he or she pretends to cry. So, the person who is telling the joke pretends to comfort the person like he or she is crying to be funny!

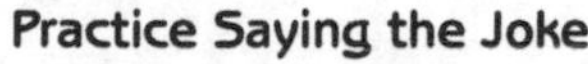

Practice Saying the Joke

Person 1: Knock knock.
Person 2: Who's there?
Person 1: Boo.
Person 2: Boo, who?
Person 1: Don't cry! It's only a joke.

REVIEW QUESTIONS: KNOCK-KNOCK JOKES

Name: ______________________________

1. You need ____ people to tell knock-knock jokes.
   A. One
   B. Two
   C. Six

2. In knock-knock jokes, the first person pretends to be knocking on a _____ .
   A. Door
   B. Wall
   C. Car

3. What does the word "Lettuce" sound like to make the joke funny?
   Person 1: Knock knock.
   Person 2: Who's there?
   Person 1: Lettuce.
   Person 2: Lettuce, who?
   Person 1: Lettuce in!
   A. Lace
   B. Iceberg
   C. Let us

4. What else in this joke is funny to think about?
   A. Salad dressing
   B. Lettuce does not talk/knock
   C. Lettuce is green

5. What was your favorite joke today?

Knock-Knock Jokes Review Questions Answer Key

1. B
2. A
3. C
4. B
5. No wrong answer

CHAPTER 10

Three W Questions of Being Funny

Lesson 1: What Is Funny?

Objectives

The participant may:

- Improve his or her understanding of what is funny vs. offensive
- Improve his or her understanding of the benefits of being funny
- Improve his or her understanding of the consequences of being offensive

Background

Explicit instruction is a research-based strategy for improving social skills for individuals with an autism spectrum disorder or other developmental disability that causes limitations of social participation (Braun et al., 2017). In this lesson, explicit instruction is used to explain what is funny vs. what is offensive, as well as the benefits and consequences of using each, respectively. Basic facial expressions are reviewed in order to help participants identify when the person is enjoying the humorous activity. Basic role-playing activities are also used, which is a valuable tool for developing social skills for individuals with autism and other developmental disabilities (Ozen et al., 2012).

Materials

- What Is Funny? Visual Story
- Review Questions and Answer Key
- What Is Funny? Sorting Cards
- Funny/Not Funny Sorting Boards

Chaiet, R. *What's So Funny?: Humor-Based Activities for Social Skill Development* (pp. 171-196).

Preparation

- Use the book or photocopy and staple together the visual story entitled What Is Funny?
- Photocopy Review Questions, one for each participant
- Photocopy and cut out What Is Funny? Sorting Cards (can be laminated to increase durability)
- Photocopy and cut out Funny/Not Funny Sorting Boards (can be laminated to increase durability)

Procedure

- Read the visual story to the participants or have them take turns reading each page. When there are questions, be sure to engage the participants and allow them to answer using their specific mode of communication (speech, communication device, sign language, gestures, etc.). For participants who seem to have a good basic understanding of the concepts in this lesson, ask more challenging questions that make the material more relatable, such as, "Has someone ever done something that was annoying and not funny to you? How did that make you feel?"
- Have the participants sort cards into Funny or Not Funny using the cards and the Funny/Not Funny boards. If the activity depicted in the card is funny, have the participant practice smiling, laughing, and/or giving a high five or handshake with a peer. If the activity depicted in the card is something that is NOT funny, have the participant practice acting sad, acting mad, and/or turning away from a friend.
- Follow up the activity by having each participant answer the Review Questions, providing assistance as needed. After the participant(s) has completed the questions, the answers given can be compared with the Answer Key.
- Extension activities for this lesson could be:
  - Showing the participants video clips of funny activities vs. inappropriate activities and having them identify which is which using the Funny/Not Funny sorting boards.

References

Braun, G., Austin, C., & Ledbetter-Cho, K. (2017). *Practice guide: Explicit instruction in reading comprehension for students with autism spectrum disorder*. U.S. Department of Education, Office of Special Education Program.

Ozen, A., Batu, S., & Birkan, B. (2012). Teaching play skills to children with autism through video modeling: Small group arrangement and observational learning. *Education and Training in Autism and Developmental Disabilities, 47*(1), 84-96.

EXERCISE: WHAT IS FUNNY?

We have been talking about different activities you can do to be funny. When you do something funny, it can make you feel happy and laugh. Can you do a big belly laugh? How about a high-voice laugh? How do you laugh? Being funny makes others feel happy and laugh, too.

This person is laughing. How can you tell he is laughing?

- Relaxed eyebrows
- Crescent-shaped mouth, smiling
- Mouth open

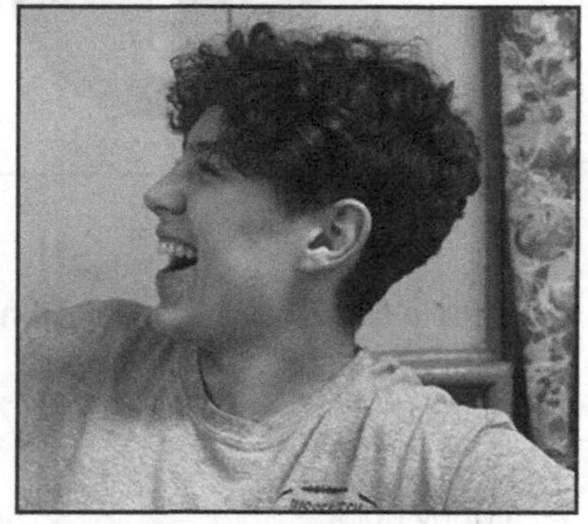

When you are funny with others, it can make them like you and want to spend time with you.

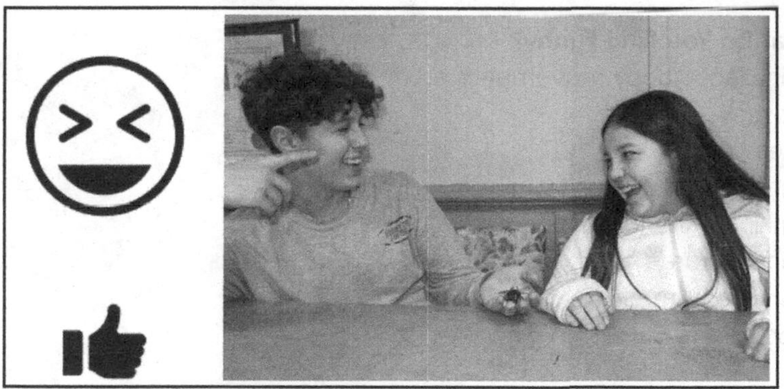

It is important to remember WHAT is funny and what is not appropriate.

People May Find Different Things Funny

- Funny faces/body movements
- Slapstick
- Jokes
- Funny noises
- Pranking a friend
- Funny pictures
- Funny costumes
- Impressions

What Do You Find Funny?

- Funny faces/body movements
- Slapstick
- Jokes
- Funny noises
- Pranking a friend
- Funny pictures
- Funny costumes
- Impressions

There are also things that we can do that are not funny.

Doing things that annoy, offend, or hurt someone is NOT funny.

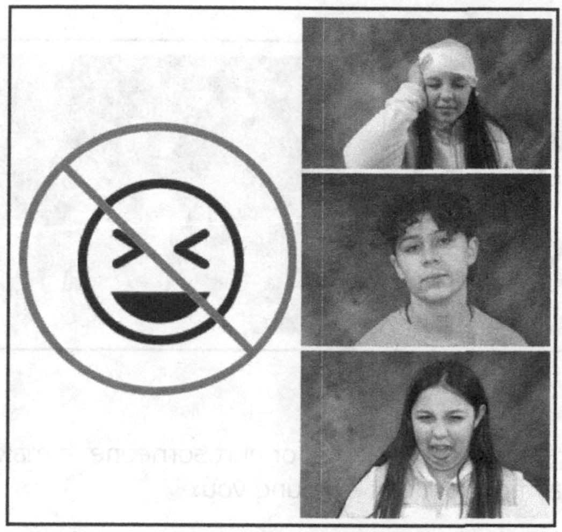

Pushing, hitting, or kicking someone is NOT funny.

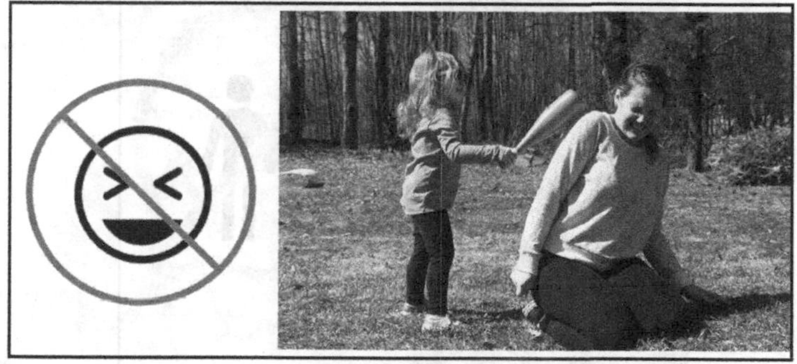

Cursing or saying things that aren't kind is NOT funny.

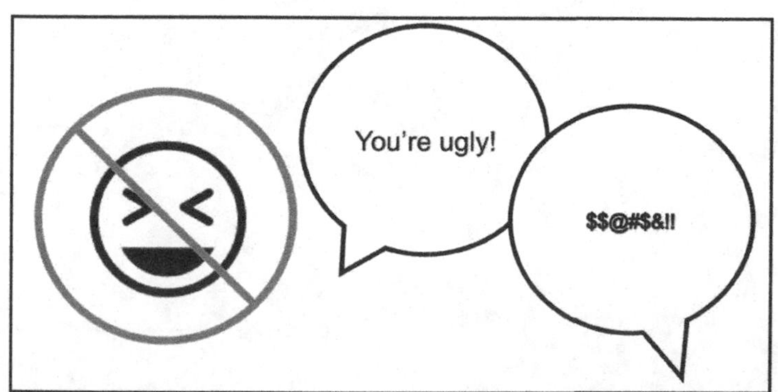

Doing jokes, pranks, or humorous activities with someone who doesn't like it is NOT funny.

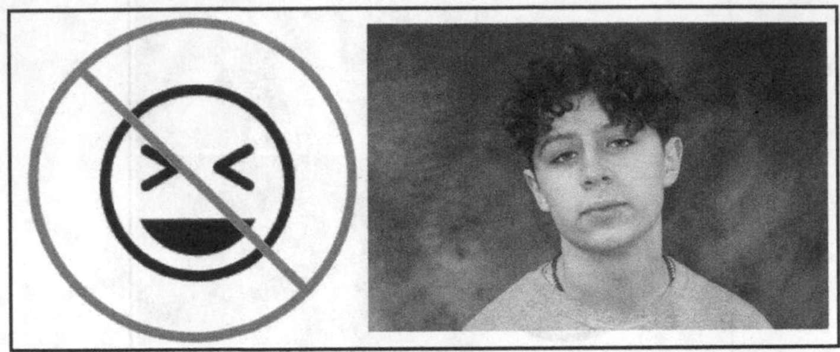

If you do things that annoy, offend, or hurt someone, it makes people sad or mad, and they may not want to be around you.

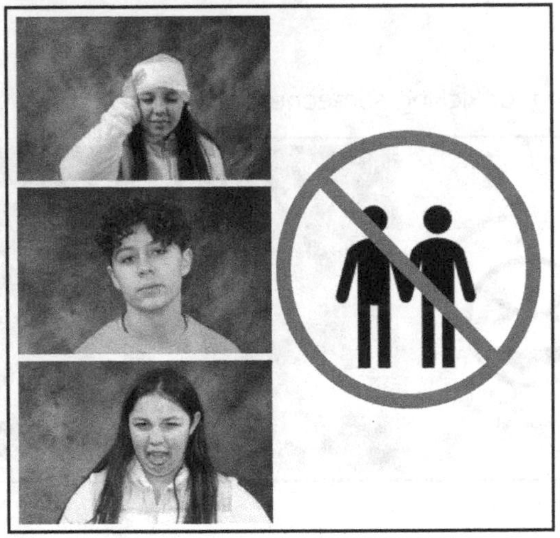

Only do things that are funny, not offensive or hurtful. This will make people like you and want to be your friend.

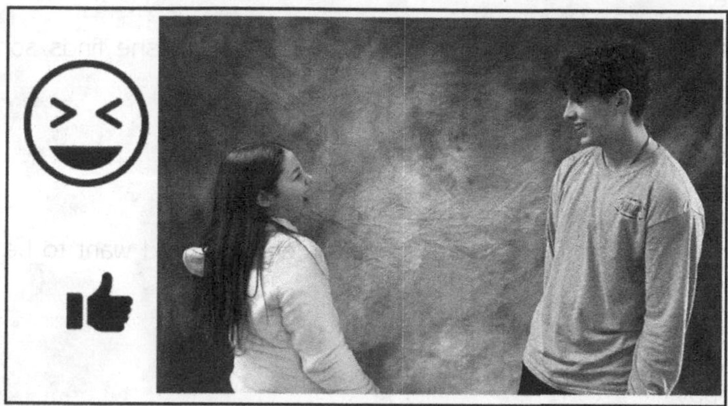

Let's Play a Game!

- Sort cards into what is funny and what is not using the Funny/Not Funny sorting boards.
- If the card says something you can use to be funny, practice smiling, laughing, and/or giving someone a high five.
- If the card says something you should not use to be funny, practice acting mad, acting sad, or turning away from someone.

REVIEW QUESTIONS: WHAT IS FUNNY?

Name:______________________________

1. Laughing is something a person does when he or she finds something ____________.
   A. Ugly
   B. Funny
   C. Mean

2. When you are funny, it makes people feel _____ and want to be around you.
   A. Mad
   B. Hurt
   C. Happy

3. Which one of these is funny?
   A. Jokes
   B. Kicking someone
   C. Yelling curse words

4. Which one of these is NOT funny?
   A. Funny faces
   B. Annoying someone
   C. Pranks

5. When you annoy, offend, or hurt someone, it makes people ______or _____ and they may not want to be around you.
   A. Sad, excited
   B. Happy, mad
   C. Sad, mad

What Is Funny? Review Questions Answer Key

1. B
2. C
3. A
4. B
5. C

Not Funny

This may make a person:

- Sad
- Mad
- NOT want to be around you

Funny

This may make a person:

- Smile
- Laugh
- Want to be around you

What Is Funny? Sorting Cards

Telling a Joke	Kicking Someone
Saying Curse Words	Playing a Prank When It Is Appropriate
Wearing Funny Costumes	Making Noises to Annoy Someone
Doing Slapstick	Saying Something Mean About Someone

Lesson 2: Who Can You Be Funny With?

Objectives

The participant may:

- Increase awareness of the emotions and personalities of others
- Improve understanding of who is and who is not appropriate to be funny with
- Improve understanding of the benefits of using humor appropriately vs. the consequences of using it inappropriately

Background

In this lesson, explicit instruction is used to explain who is appropriate to use humor with and who is not (Braun et al., 2017). The importance of being aware of a person's emotions, his or her personality, and his or her specific role before trying to be funny with him or her is discussed. By encouraging the participants to consider emotions and personality, it helps to practice the skill of being more aware of others and to understand the impact of their actions on others. Basic role-playing activities are used again, which is a valuable tool for developing social skills for individuals with autism and other intellectual disabilities (Ozen et al., 2012).

Materials

- Who Can You Be Funny With? Visual Story
- Review Questions and Answer Key
- Who Can You Be Funny With? Sorting Cards
- Funny/Not Funny Sorting Boards

Preparation

- Use the book or photocopy and staple together the visual story entitled Who Can You Be Funny With?
- Photocopy Review Questions, one for each participant
- Photocopy and cut out Who Can You Be Funny With? Sorting Cards (can be laminated to increase durability)
- Photocopy and cut out Funny/Not Funny Sorting Boards (can be laminated to increase durability)

Procedure

- Read the visual story to the participants or have them take turns reading each page. When there are questions, be sure to engage the participants and allow them to answer using their specific mode of communication (speech, communication device, sign language, gestures, etc.). For participants who seem to have a good basic understanding of the concepts in this lesson, ask more challenging questions that make the material more relatable, such as, "Do you know someone who really likes to be silly? Who is it? Do you think it is okay to be funny with a police officer when he or she is working? Why or why not?"
- Have the participants sort cards into Funny or Not Funny using the cards and the Funny/Not Funny boards. If the person depicted in the card is someone you can be funny with, have the participant practice smiling, laughing, and/or giving a high five or handshake with a peer. If the person depicted in the card is someone you should not be funny with, have the participant practice acting sad, mad, and/or turning away from a friend.
- Follow up the activity by having each participant answer the Review Questions, providing assistance as needed. After the participant(s) has completed the questions, the answers given can be compared with the Answer Key.
- Extension activities for this lesson could be:
    - Showing the participants video clips of people who are demonstrating different moods/personalities/roles and having them identify who you can be funny with and who you cannot using the Funny/Not Funny sorting boards.

References

Braun, G., Austin, C., & Ledbetter-Cho, K. (2017). *Practice guide: Explicit instruction in reading comprehension for students with autism spectrum disorder*. U.S. Department of Education, Office of Special Education Program.

Ozen, A., Batu, S., & Birkan, B. (2012). Teaching play skills to children with autism through video modeling: Small group arrangement and observational learning. *Education and Training in Autism and Developmental Disabilities*, *47*(1), 84-96.

EXERCISE: WHO CAN YOU BE FUNNY WITH?

Today, we are going to talk about WHO you can be funny with. If you are funny with some people, it will make them happy and enjoy spending time with you.

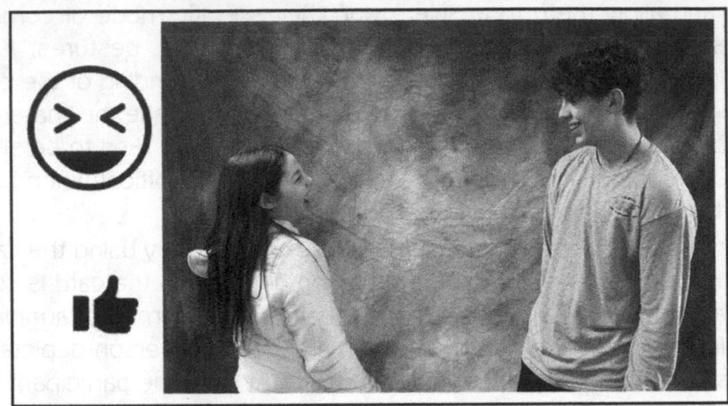

Other people may not be happy if you are funny with them. It might make them feel sad or mad, and they may not want to be around you.

One thing you should think about before you are funny with someone is the way a person is feeling. If a person is feeling happy or excited, you can be funny with him or her.

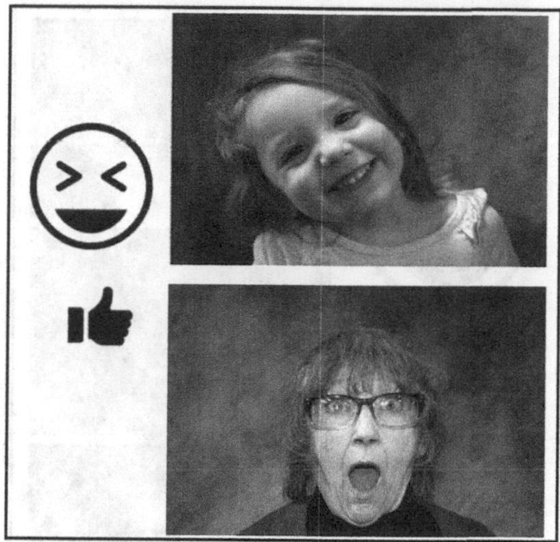

If a person is feeling mad or sad, you should not be funny with them. It may make him or her more upset.

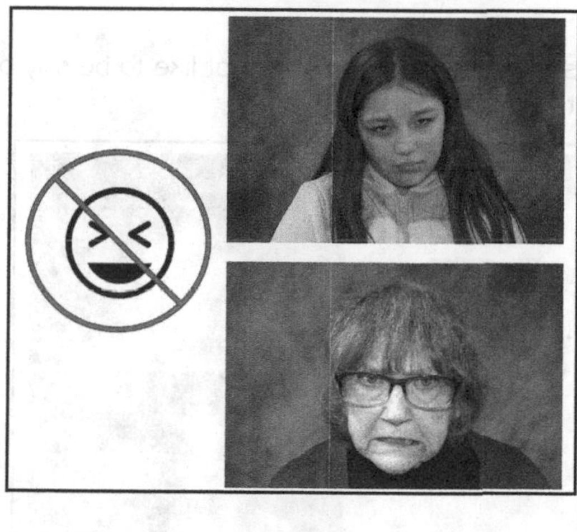

You should also think about a person's personality before you are funny with him or her. If the person is a silly and likes to joke around and have fun, you can be funny with him or her.

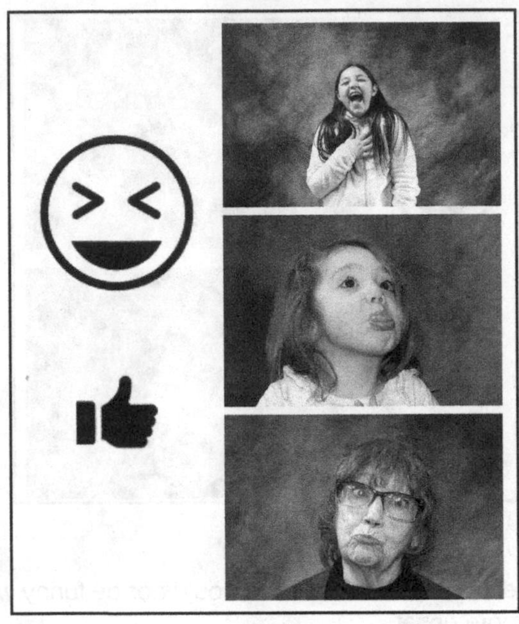

If the person is more serious and does not like to be silly often, you should not be funny with them.

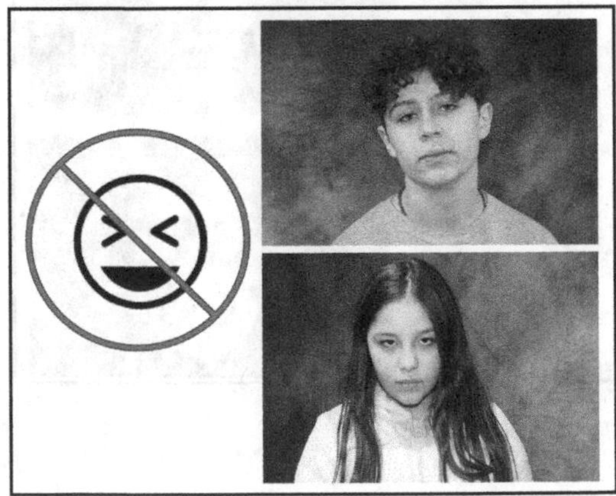

You should also think about a person's job and how you know him or her.

If the person is a friend, family member, or someone else you know well, you can be funny with him or her.

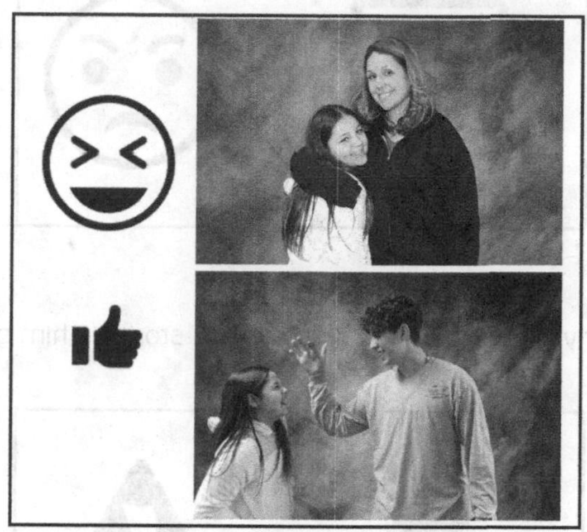

If the person has an important job to do, like a teacher or a firefighter, you should not interrupt his or her job to be funny with him or her.

If you are funny with a teacher when he or she is teaching, he or she may be upset because the teacher is trying to teach the class.

If you are funny with a firefighter, you may be stopping him or her from keeping people safe.

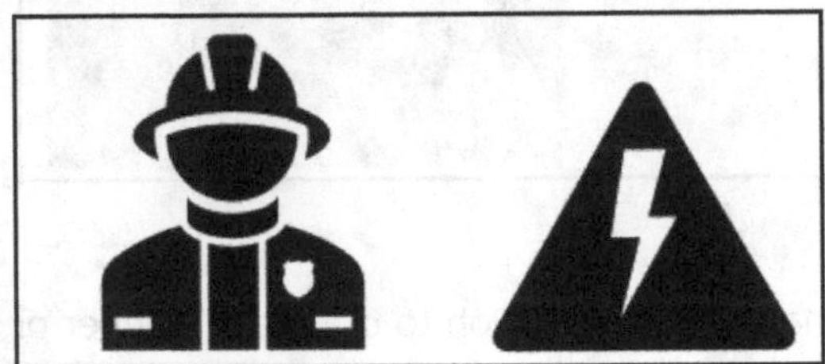

Only be funny with the right people, and it will make him or her happy and enjoy spending time with you.

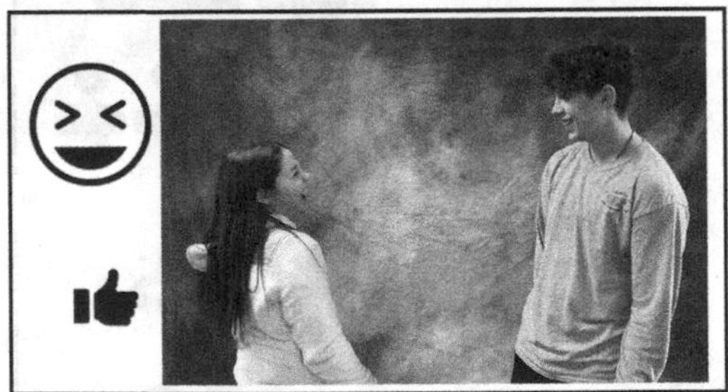

Let's Play a Game!

- Sort cards into who you can and cannot be funny with using the Funny/Not Funny sorting boards.
- If the card says a person you can be funny with, practice smiling, laughing, and/or giving someone a high five.
- If the card says someone you should not be funny with, practice acting mad, acting sad, or turning away from someone.

REVIEW QUESTIONS: WHO CAN YOU BE FUNNY WITH?

Name: ______________________________

1. If a person is feeling happy/excited, you __________ be funny with them.
   A. Should not
   B. Cannot
   C. Can

2. If you are funny with a person who is feeling mad, it may make them more __________.
   A. Upset
   B. Happy
   C. Fun

3. Should you be funny with this person?
   A. Yes
   B. No

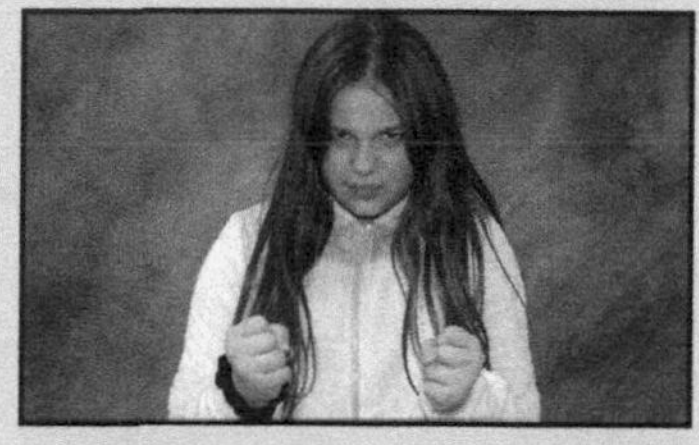

4. Should you be funny with this person?
   A. Yes
   B. No

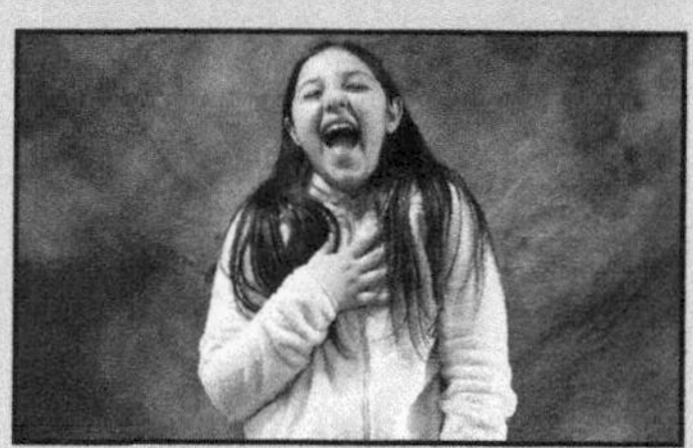

5. Should you be funny with a firefighter?
   A. Yes
   B. No

Who Can You Be Funny With?
Review Questions Answer Key

1. C
2. A
3. B
4. A
5. B

Who Can You Be Funny With? Sorting Cards

Silly Person	Mad Mood
Happy Mood	Serious Person
Firefighter	Excited Mood
Teacher	Sad Mood

Lesson 3: When Can You Be Funny?

Objectives

The participant may:

- Increase awareness of appropriate vs. inappropriate times to use humor
- Improve understanding of the benefits of using humor appropriately vs. the consequences of using it inappropriately

Background

This lesson uses explicit instruction to discuss the appropriate time and place to use humor (Braun et al., 2017). Social narratives, like the one used in this lesson, can be very effective in helping individuals with developmental disabilities understand and observe pro-social behavior in specific environments (Karayazi et al., 2014). This visual lesson describes which times and environments are not acceptable or even unsafe to be funny in and gives a brief description of why this is the case. This instruction can help individuals with disabilities be more successful in various community settings. Once again, basic role-playing activities are used, which is a valuable tool for developing social skills for individuals with autism and other intellectual disabilities (Ozen et al., 2012).

Materials

- When Can You Be Funny? Visual Story
- Review Questions and Answer Key
- When Can You Be Funny? Sorting Cards
- Funny/Not Funny Sorting Boards

Preparation

- Use the book or photocopy and staple together the visual story entitled When Can You Be Funny?
- Photocopy Review Questions, one for each participant
- Photocopy and cut out When Can You Be Funny? Sorting Cards (can be laminated to increase durability)
- Photocopy and cut out Funny/Not Funny Sorting Boards (can be laminated to increase durability)

Procedure

- Read the visual story to the participants or have them take turns reading each page. When there are questions, be sure to engage the participants and allow them to answer using their specific mode of communication (speech, communication device, sign language, gestures, etc.). For participants who seem to have a good basic understanding of the concepts in this lesson, ask more challenging questions that make the material more relatable, such as, "Is there a good time at school to be funny? Is there a good time at home to be funny? What are these times?"
- Have the participants sort cards into Funny or Not Funny using the cards and the Funny/Not Funny boards. If the activity depicted in the card is a good time to be funny, have the participant practice smiling, laughing, and/or giving a high five or handshake with a peer. If the activity depicted in the card is not a good time to be funny, have the participant practice acting sad, acting mad, and/or turning away from a friend.
- Follow up the activity by having each participant answer the Review Questions, providing assistance as needed. After the participant(s) has completed the questions, the answers given can be compared with the Answer Key.
- Extension activities for this lesson could be:
  - Showing the participants video clips or photographs of various environments and times of the day and having them identify when you can be funny and when you cannot using the Funny/Not Funny sorting boards.

References

Braun, G., Austin, C., & Ledbetter-Cho, K. (2017). *Practice guide: Explicit instruction in reading comprehension for students with autism spectrum disorder*. U.S. Department of Education, Office of Special Education Program.

Karayazi, S., Evans, P., & Filer, J. (2014). The effects of a Social Story intervention on the pro-social behaviors of a young adult with autism spectrum disorder. *International Journal of Special Education, 29*(3), 126-133.

Ozen, A., Batu, S., & Birkan, B. (2012). Teaching play skills to children with autism through video modeling: Small group arrangement and observational learning. *Education and Training in Autism and Developmental Disabilities, 47*(1), 84-96.

EXERCISE: WHEN CAN YOU BE FUNNY?

Today, we are going to talk about WHEN you can be funny. If you are funny at the right times, people will be happy and ready to laugh with you.

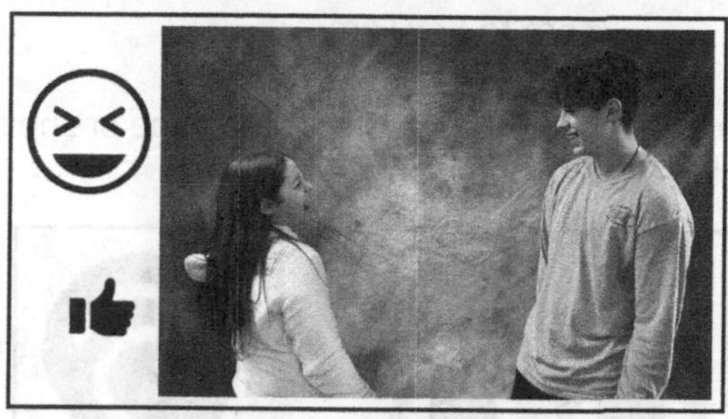

If you are funny at the wrong time, people will not be ready to laugh with you. They may be mad or annoyed that you are interrupting them from important things they are doing.

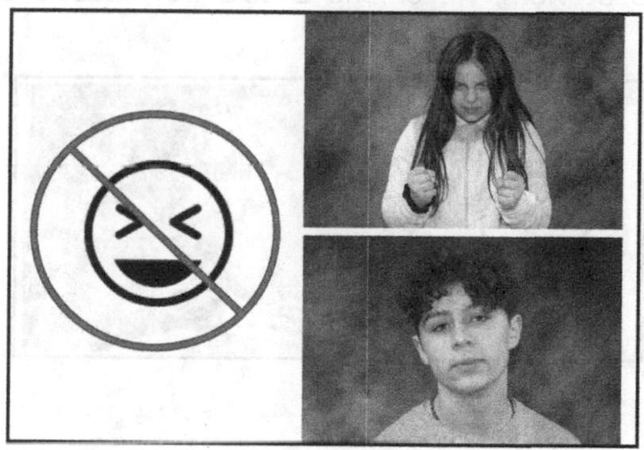

If you are funny at the wrong time, you may also be stopping yourself from doing what you are supposed to be. Different times of the day are for different activities.

School/Work	8 am to 3 pm
Dinner	5 pm
Free Time	6 pm to 8:30 pm

You only want to be funny at the times of the day when there is not something else happening, like during "free time":

School/Work	8 am to 3 pm
Dinner	5 pm
Free Time	6 pm to 8:30 pm

If a person is in the middle of a lesson at school, he or she should be sitting, looking, and listening—NOT being funny.

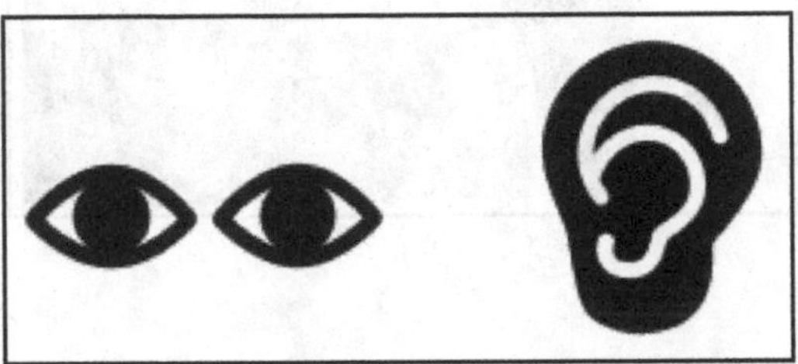

If a person is at work, he or she should be focused on doing work—NOT being funny.

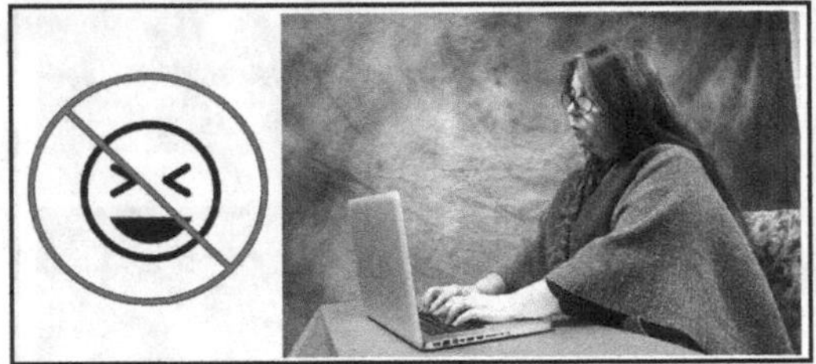

During a movie, play, or religious service, you should be sitting, looking, and listening—NOT being funny.

If you and a family member both have free time at home, it is the perfect time to be funny.

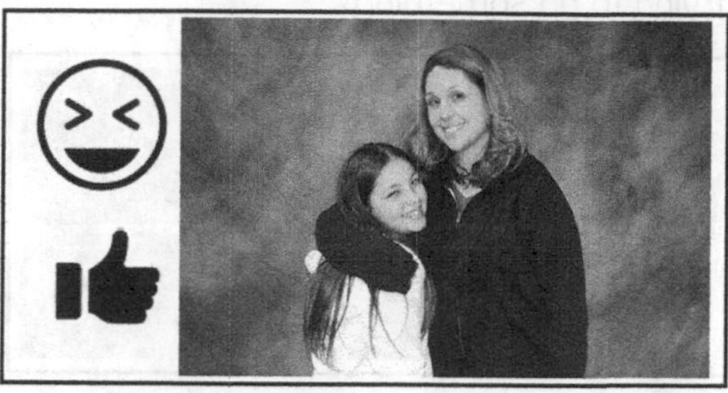

If you and a friend or co-worker have recess or break during school/work, it is the perfect time to be funny.

- School
- Work
- Science
- Arrive at work
- Math
- **Break/Lunch**
- **Recess**
- Leave work

There are some times that are unsafe to be funny, such as during a real emergency or fire drill. This means that if you try to be funny, it may put you or another person in danger. You may also get in trouble.

It is important that the people you are being funny with are ALSO not busy! Even if it is a good time for you to be funny, you do not want to bother other people if they are trying to do something.

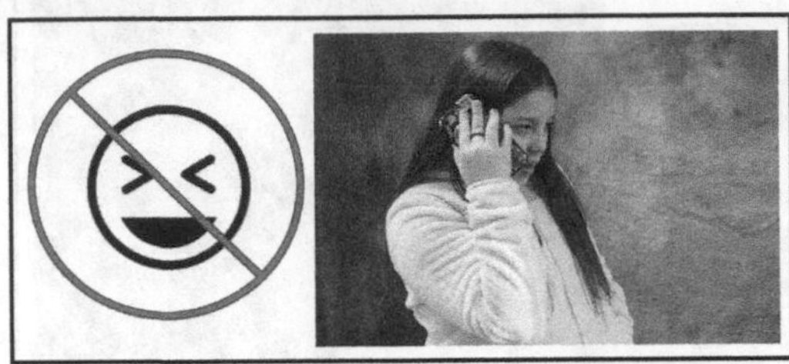

Only be funny at the right times, and people will be happy and ready to laugh with you.

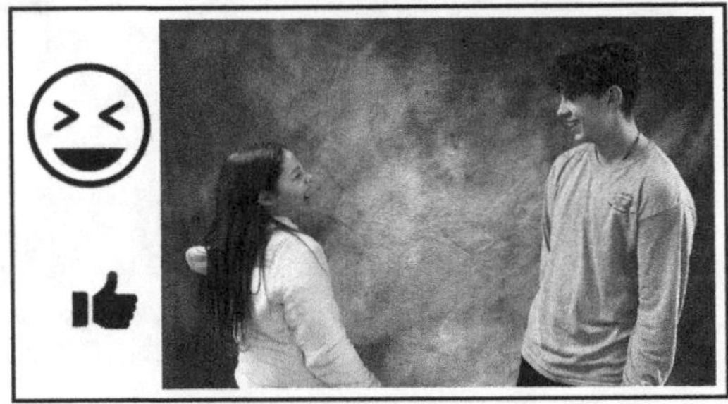

REVIEW QUESTIONS: WHEN CAN YOU BE FUNNY?

Name:______________________________

1. There are good times to be funny and bad times to be funny.
   A. True
   B. False

2. When is a good time to be funny?
   A. Religious service
   B. Free time
   C. At work

3. When is it unsafe to be funny?
   A. During free time at home
   B. During break time at work
   C. During an emergency

4. If you are funny at the right times, it makes people feel ________.
   A. Mad
   B. Happy
   C. Sad

5. During lesson at school, you should be sitting, looking, and ________.
   A. Listening
   B. Yelling
   C. Crying

When Can You Be Funny?
Review Questions Answer Key

1. A
2. B
3. C
4. B
5. A

When Can You Be Funny? Sorting Cards

Break at Work	Fire Drill
Free Time at Home	When a Friend Is on the Phone
Recess at School	During Lesson at School
Religious Service	While at Work

Index

animals, funny, 79-80
background, 79
cow, 81
dog, 82
exercises, 81-85
fish, 83
materials, 80
objectives, 79
preparation, 80
procedure, 80
review, 86
spider, 84
audience, 1

baby, funny, 89
background, 5-8
developmental disabilities, individuals with, 7
humor development, 6-7
order of lessons, 5
social-emotional development, 5-6
teaching humor, 7
benefits, overview, 2
"Big Sneeze" expression, 22-23
body, funny, 26-27
background, 26
exercises, 28-32
materials, 26
objectives, 26
preparation, 26
procedure, 27
review, 33
bug pranks, 111-112
background, 111
exercises, 113-115
fly in a drink prank, 113
materials, 111
objectives, 111
preparation, 111
procedure, 112
review, 116
rolling cockroach prank, 114
spider on a string prank, 115

car, funny sizes, 99
chips prank, 103
clown costume, 37
costume hat, 38

costumes, funny, 35-36
  activities, 41-43
  background, 35
  clowns, 37
  costume hat, 38
  crazy outfit, 42
  exercises, 37-40
  funny glasses, 39
  funny hair, 39
  funny hats, 41
  funny neckwear, 40
  glasses, 41
  halloween costumes, 37
  materials, 36
  neckwear, 42
  objectives, 35
  preparation, 36
  procedure, 36
  review, 43
  sports team mascots, 37
  wigs, 41
cow, funny, 81
cowboy impressions, 46-50
crazy outfit, 42

development
  of humor, 6-7
  social-emotional, 5-6
developmental disabilities, individuals with, 7
dog, funny, 82
dog poop prank, 119
dollar on a string prank, 125

exercises, review, 170
expressions, 35-43

face, funny, 9-11
  acting, 19-20
    background, 19
    "Big Sneeze," 22-23
    exercises, 21-24
    materials, 19
    objectives, 19
    preparation, 19
    procedure, 20
    review, 25
    "Stinky Sock," 21-22
    "Wake up," 23-24
  background, 9
  exercises, 12-16
  materials, 10
  name that emotion, 17
    cards, 17
  objectives, 9
  preparation, 10
  procedure, 10-11
  review, 18
fish, funny, 83
fly in a drink prank, 113
food pranks, 101-102
  background, 101
  chips prank, 103
  exercises, 103-104
  ice cream popper prank, 104
  materials, 101
  objectives, 101
  preparation, 102
  procedure, 102
  review, 105
funny animals, 79-80
  background, 79
  cow, 81
  dog, 82
  exercises, 81-85
  fish, 83
  materials, 80
  objectives, 79
  preparation, 80
  procedure, 80
  review, 86
  spider, 84

funny body, 26-27
- background, 26
- exercises, 28-32
- materials, 26
- objectives, 26
- preparation, 26
- procedure, 27
- review, 33

funny glasses, 39
funny hair, 39
funny hats, 41
funny neckwear, 40
funny people, 87-88
- baby, 89
- background, 87
- exercises, 89-92
- materials, 87
- objectives, 87
- older lady, 90
- preparation, 87
- procedure, 88
- review, 93

funny sizes, 94-95
- background, 94
- car, 99
- exercises, 96-99
- glasses, 97
- hands, 97
- hats, 97-98
- materials, 94
- nose, 97
- objectives, 94
- preparation, 94
- procedure, 95
- review, 100
- shoes, 96
- umbrella, 98

glasses, 41
- funny, 39
- funny sizes, 97

gross pranks, 117-118
- background, 117
- dog poop prank, 119
- exercises, 119-120
- materials, 117
- objectives, 117
- preparation, 117
- procedure, 118
- review, 121
- whoopee cushion prank, 120

hair, funny, 39
halloween costumes, 37
hands, funny sizes, 97
hats
- funny, 41
- funny sizes, 97-98

homophone jokes, 150-151
- background, 150
- exercises, 152-155
- materials, 150
- objectives, 150
- preparation, 150
- procedure, 151
- review, 156

humor development, 6-7
humor habits program, overview, 3

ice cream popper prank, 104
impressions, 44-45
- background, 44
- cowboy, 46-50
- exercises, 46-51
- materials, 44
- objectives, 44
- preparation, 44
- princess, 46-49, 51
- procedure, 45
- review, 52
- superhero, 46-49, 51
- zombie, 46-50

incongruency, 79-100
funny animals, 79-80. *See also* funny animals
funny people, 87-88. *See also* funny people
funny sizes, 94-95
instruction, overview, 2
intended participants, 1-2

jokes, 143-170
homophone jokes, 150-151. *See also* homophone jokes
knock-knock jokes, 164-165. *See also* knock-knock jokes
rhyming jokes, 143-170. *See also* rhyming jokes
silly sound jokes, 157-158. *See also* silly sound jokes

knock-knock jokes, 164-165
background, 164
exercises, 166-169
materials, 164
objectives, 164
preparation, 164
procedure, 165

messy slapstick, 65-66
activities, 69-77
background, 65
exercises, 67-68
materials, 65
objectives, 65
preparation, 66
procedure, 66
review, 78
money pranks, 122-123
background, 122
dollar on a string prank, 125
exercises, 124-126
materials, 122
objectives, 122
preparation, 122
procedure, 123
review, 127
rolling coin prank, 126
stuck coin prank, 124
motor planning exercises, 3
overview, 3

name that emotion, 17
cards, 17
neckwear, 42
funny, 40
nose, funny sizes, 97

older lady, funny, 90
order of lessons, 5
overview
audience, 1
benefits, 2
humor habits program, 3
instruction, 2
intended participants, 1-2
social interaction, 3
strategies, 2-3

people, funny, 87-88
baby, 89
background, 87
exercises, 89-92
materials, 87
objectives, 87
older lady, 90
preparation, 87
procedure, 88
review, 93
persons with whom to be funny, 180-181
background, 180
exercises, 182-186
materials, 180

objectives, 180
preparation, 180
procedure, 181
review, 187-188
physical comedy, 9-34
body, 26-33. *See also* body
costumes, 35-52. *See also* costumes
expressions, 35-43. *See also* expressions
face, 9-25. *See also* face
impressions, 44-45. *See also* impressions
slapstick, 53-78. *See also* slapstick
pranks, 101-128
bug pranks, 111-112. *See also* bug pranks
food pranks, 101-102. *See also* food pranks
gross pranks, 117-118. *See also* gross pranks
money pranks, 122-123. *See also* money pranks
water pranks, 106-107. *See also* water pranks
princess impressions, 46-49, 51

question-and-answer jokes, 145
questions
funny, defining, 171-172
timing, 189-190
with whom, 180-181

rhyming jokes, 143-170
background, 143
exercises, 145-148
materials, 143
objectives, 143
preparation, 144
procedure, 144
question-and-answer jokes, 145
review, 149
rhyming words, 135-136
background, 135
exercises, 137-140
materials, 135
objectives, 135
preparation, 135
procedure, 136
review, 141
rolling cockroach prank, 114
rolling coin prank, 126

shoes, funny sizes, 96
silly sound jokes, 157-158
background, 157
exercises, 159-162
materials, 157
objectives, 157
preparation, 157
procedure, 158
review, 163
sizes, funny, 94-95
background, 94
car, 99
exercises, 96-99
glasses, 97
hands, 97
hats, 97-98
materials, 94
nose, 97
objectives, 94
preparation, 94
procedure, 95
review, 100
shoes, 96
umbrella, 98
slapstick, 53-78
activities, 56-63
background, 53
exercises, 55
introduction to, 53-54
materials, 54

messy slapstick, 65-66
activities, 69-77
background, 65
exercises, 67-68
materials, 65
objectives, 65
preparation, 66
procedure, 66
review, 78
objectives, 53
preparation, 54
procedure, 54
review, 64
social-emotional development, 5-6
social interaction, 3
sound effects, 129-130, 133
background, 129
exercises, 131-133
materials, 130
objectives, 129
preparation, 130
procedure, 130
review, 134
sound play, 129-130
sound effects, 129-130. *See also* sound effects
spider, funny, 84
spider on a string prank, 115
sports team mascots, 37
squirting flower prank, 109
squirting ring prank, 108
"Stinky Sock" expression, 21-22
strategies, overview, 2-3
stuck coin prank, 124
superhero impressions, 46-49, 51

teaching humor, 7

umbrella, funny sizes, 98

"Wake up" expression, 23-24
water pranks, 106-107
background, 106
exercises, 108-109
materials, 106
objectives, 106
preparation, 106
procedure, 107
review, 110
squirting flower prank, 109
squirting ring prank, 108
what is funny?, 171-172
background, 171
exercises, 173-177
materials, 171
objectives, 171
preparation, 172
procedure, 172
review, 178-179
when can you be funny?, 189-190
background, 189
exercises, 191-194
materials, 189
objectives, 189
preparation, 189
procedure, 190
review, 195-196
whoopee cushion prank, 120
wigs, 41
word play, 131-142
rhyming words, 131-142. *See also* rhyming words

zombie impressions, 46-50

Printed in the United States
by Baker & Taylor Publisher Services